AF844147

Diana K. Reese

Reproducing Enlightenment

Interdisciplinary German Cultural Studies

Edited by
Scott Denham · Irene Kacandes
Jonathan Petropoulos

Volume 5

Walter de Gruyter · Berlin · New York

Diana K. Reese

Reproducing Enlightenment: Paradoxes in the Life of the Body Politic

Literature and Philosophy around 1800

W DE G

Walter de Gruyter · Berlin · New York

♾ Printed on acid-free paper which falls within the guidelines
of the ANSI to ensure permanence and durability.

Library of Congress Cataloging-in-Publication Data

A CIP catalogue record for this book is available from the Library of Congress.

ISBN 978-3-11-020600-5
ISSN 1861-8030

Bibliographic information published by the Deutsche Nationalbibliothek

The Deutsche Nationalbibliothek lists this publication in the Deutsche Nationalbibliografie; detailed bibliographic data are available in the Internet at http://dnb.d-nb.de.

© Copyright 2009 by Walter de Gruyter GmbH & Co. KG, 10785 Berlin,
www.degruyter.com
All rights reserved, including those of translation into foreign languages. No parts of this book may be reproduced in any form or by any means, electronic or mechanical, including photocopy, recording, or any information storage and retrieval system, without permission in writing from the publisher.

Printed in Germany

Image, page v: 'Reading the Iliad', copyright K. Anaid Eseer, 1983
Cover design: Christopher Schneider, Berlin
Printing and binding: Hubert & Co. GmbH & Co. KG, Göttingen

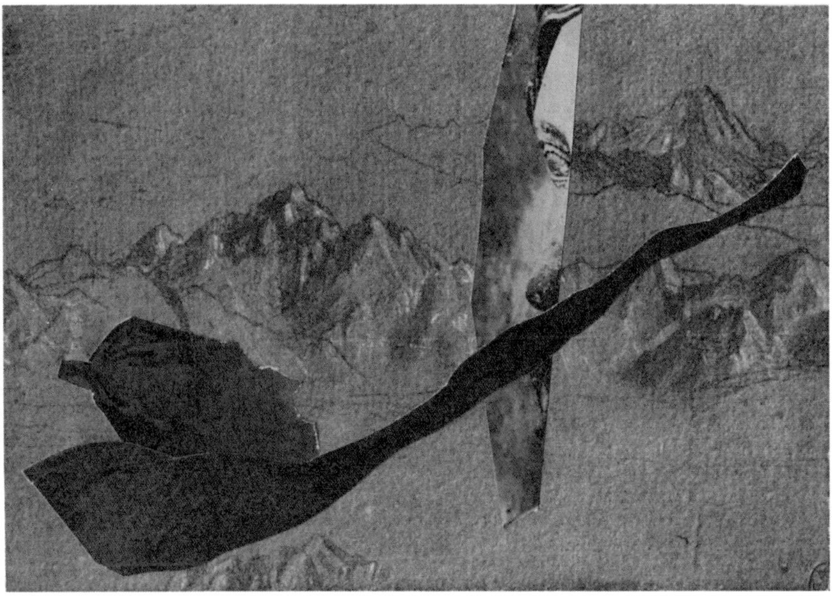

That story is not true
You never sailed in the benched ships
You never went to the city of Troy.
– Stesichorus

Acknowledgments

I would like to thank the *Stiftung des Abgeordnetenhauses, Berlin*, for a generous grant that allowed me to dedicate a year of research in Berlin to this project and the journal *Representations* for choosing to publish an earlier version of my work on *Frankenstein: A Modern Prometheus* and permitting me to reprint passages here which first appeared in their journal. I am happily indebted to my many teachers over the years for inspiring me with their eloquence and for the gift of their time, intelligence and creativity, especially: Rose Sleigh, Dee Frank, Wai-Lim Yip, Dalia Judovitz, Padmanabh Jaini, Avital Ronell, Andreas Huyssen, Dorothea von Mücke, Deborah White and Gayatri Chakravorty Spivak. I would like to express my warm gratitude to Irene Kacandes for her careful reading, thoughtful commentary and extremely generous correspondence throughout the editing of this book. I thank Kent Steinriede and Lisa Bhattarcharji for their painstaking work as copy-editors, Andreas Brandmair, Christine Henschel and Michael Peschke for providing indispensable help with the formatting, copy-editing and preparation of the final manuscript and Manuela Gerlof for her incredible patience and steadying contribution to bringing this book to press. Laura Rubinstein, Joan Filler, Jeanette Palmer and Robyn Priti Ross offered their dedication and support to the very possibility of this work. I would like to take this opportunity to thank friends, teachers, students and colleagues – some all at once – who have offered so much encouragement and given energy to this project through imaginative, revitalizing conversation: Leslie Adelson, David Bathrick, Madeleine Reich-Casad, Joshua Dittrich, Donald Downs, Peter Gilgen, Peter Hohendahl, Taran Kang, Richard Korb, Joseph Lemelin, Gunhild Lischke, Tracy McNulty, Natalie Melas, Keyzom Ngodup, Martin Puchner, Eric Rentschler, Zhanna Rosenberg, Anette Schwarz and Geoffrey Waite. I recall in gratitude my family, my brother, Peter Winter Reese, and my parents Warren Paul and Kathryn Anne who first taught me a love of words. Neither this book, nor I, would exist if not for my friends, teachers themselves of the finest kind, who call out from the other shore, "Stay afloat, head out, come across!" Elizabeth Akerman, Cathy Lee Crane, Holiday Dapper, Dallas Denery, Robert Fitzpatrick, Michael Gotkin, Matthew Hartman, Andreas Kleiser, Hildegard Kleiser, Benjamin Lane, Daniel Leonard, Carin McLain, Chris Mills, Nick Mullner, Kirsten

Painter, Natassa Papadede, Lecia Rosenthal, Andrew Rubin, Yvette Siegert, Kent Steinriede, Dominique Treilhou, Dorothea von Moltke and Lindsey Smith Welcome. May you ever find the time to read what you have wrought!

Table of Contents

Introduction

> Ruthless toward itself, the Enlightenment has eradicated the last remnant of its own self-awareness. Only thought that does violence to itself is hard enough to shatter myths.
> – Theodor W. Adorno and Max Horkheimer

In the 1944 Preface to their *Dialectic of Enlightenment*, Theodor W. Adorno and Max Horkheimer take up a position one would be more apt to associate with Ernst Bloch: that in the face of enlightenment's self-annihilation as myth, enlightenment must look to fulfill past hopes.[1]

> … die Aufklärung muß sich auf sich selbst besinnen, wenn die Menschen nicht vollends verraten werden sollen. Nicht um die Konservierung der Vergangenheit, sondern um die Einlösung der vergangenen Hoffnung ist es zu tun.

> … enlightenment must reflect on itself if humanity is not to be totally betrayed. What is at stake is not conservation of the past but the fulfillment (Einlösung) of past hopes. (Translation modified.)

The operative figure of fulfillment (*Einlösung*) here is economic and not soteriological. It verges on "redemption" – but only in the sense that one redeems the deposit on a bottle. Adorno and Horkheimer do not tarry long with this positive assertion, however, for the very next sentence lands us straight in the crux of the dilemma: "Today, however, the past is being continued as destruction of the past." (xvii) (*Heute aber setzt die Vergangenheit sich fort als Zerstörung der Vergangenheit.*) The preservation of culture as a value only further assures the obliteration of enlightenment's hope to elude domination and fear.

Interestingly, in the demand they raise for a persistent possibility in reflection – "enlightenment must reflect on itself" – Adorno and Horkheimer undertake the challenge of providing a positive concept:

1 Max Horkheimer and Theodor W. Adorno, *Dialektik der Aufklärung: Philosophische Fragmente* (Frankfurt a.M.: Fischer Verlag, 1994), 5. English: Max Horkheimer and Theodor W. Adorno, *Dialectic of Enlightenment: Philosophical Fragments*, trans. Edmund Jephcott (Stanford: Stanford University Press, 2002), xvii. Hereafter cited in text as *DA* or *DE* with page numbers in parentheses.

> Die dabei an Aufklärung geübte Kritik soll einen positiven Begriff von ihr vorbereiten, der sie aus ihrer Verstrickung in blinder Herrschaft löst. (*DA*, 6)
>
> The critique of enlightenment given in this section is intended to prepare a positive concept of enlightenment which liberates it from its entanglement in blind domination. (*DE*, xviii)

While working largely to unveil the ruse of the positive concept of experience fostered by enlightenment critique, their treatment should nonetheless yield a positive concept of enlightenment. The critique thus also addresses the endurance of unreflected enlightenment precepts in socialist modes of analysis: Adorno and Horkheimer's polemic is not only leveled at the consumer capitalist leviathan (as which it is so often remembered) but also describes the futility of the praxis that attempts to challenge it.[2]

> Indem er [der Socialist] für alle Zukunft die Notwendigkeit zur Basis erhob und den Geist auf gut idealistisch zur höchsten Spitze depravierte, hielt er das Erbe der bürgerlichen Philosophie allzu krampfhaft fest ... Umwälzende wahre Praxis aber hängt ab von der Unnachgiebigkeit der Theorie gegen die Bewußtlosigkeit, mit der die Gesellschaft das Denken sich verhärten läßt. (*DA*, 48)
>
> In declaring necessity the sole basis of the future and banishing mind, in the best idealist fashion, to the far pinnacle of the superstructure, socialism clung all too desperately to the heritage of bourgeois philosophy… But a true praxis capable of overturning the staus quo depends on theory's refusal to yield to the oblivion in which society allows thought to ossify. (*DE*, 32-33)

Writing in exile in Los Angeles during the second world war, Adorno and Horkheimer make an unusual move toward a positive concept, an affirmation of sorts, to break the impasse from which their work sets out: the self-destruction of enlightenment understood not only as a failed hope but also as one forgotten.

Living on through the survival of cultural institutions – that is to say, conditions in which thought appears as commodity and language its celebration – this book considers the endurance of a figure which haunts the presentation of enlightenment at the level of its concept: reproduction. For if critique of enlightenment is long-since practiced as the correct an-

---

2 "Der mythische wissenschaftliche Respekt der Völker vor dem Gegebenen, das sie doch immerzu schaffen, wird schließlich selbst zur positiven Tatsache, zur Zwingburg, der gegenüber noch die revolutionäre Phantasie sich als Utopismus vor sich selber sich schämt und zum fügsamen Vertrauen auf die objektive Tendenz der Geschichte entartet." (*DA*, 48). "….The mythical scientific respect of peoples for the given reality, which they themselves constantly create, finally becomes itself a positive fact, a fortress before which even the revolutionary imagination feels shamed as utopianism, and degenerates to a compliant trust in the objective tendency of history." (*DE*, 33)

swer in an entrance exam, its study has settled down into a continuation of the work generated by Adorno and Horkheimer's critique sometimes at the expense of their barely sketched hope. If enlightenment cancels itself in its collapse with the fatality of the mythic, it persists fatally where it is precomprehended as a given under a historicist rubric. In order to stay attuned to the "event" of the Enlightenment as something destroyed in its coming to pass, one must still attend to its liminal status as that which becomes history through its very conceptual production thereof. Thus enlightenment is currently reproduced *both* as determinate local and historical era subject to critique *and* as a regulatory ideal proffered in ambitions for international governance. As contingent instance it becomes unreflected, as transhistorical it falls to its own logic. The student of the Enlightenment thus passes through Adorno and Horkheimer's work as both compulsory and, in the never-lost name of progress, superceded. Whether as era or idea, enlightenment as object of study faces the threat of its own reproduction.

In the antithesis Adorno and Horkheimer propose:

> ... schon der Mythos ist Aufklärung, und Aufklärung schlägt in Mythologie zurück. (*DA*, 6)

> ... Myth is already enlightenment, and enlightenment reverts to mythology. (*DE*, xviii)

the question of repetition and reproduction grounds the identity-in-negation of each term in the chiasmus. Mythology vainly attempts to master nature through mimetic repetition, whereas enlightenment *actually* masters through an experimental reproducibility that consigns both its agent and its other to loss (labor and mastery in mechanization). In both instances, a barren repetition makes for the dilemma. Indeed, the thought of some fruition *beyond* repetition offers the argument rhetorical force, alerting us that an old domestic problem lingers on in "reproduction" as the eclipsed but necessary term of the critique.

Reproduction, as the issue that can link mimesis, the other key term in the analysis, to both the mythic and the enlightenment modes, haunts the critical subject of knowledge as both its precondition and the threat of its dissolution.[3] The first indication of the importance of this figure of repro-

---

3 Here I refer specifically to Louis Althusser's use of the term in his essay on ideological state apparatuses: every social formation must not only reproduce the conditions of production, but also *the existing relations of production.* Althusser's theorization of the materiality of this reproduction as "practices" allows him to include under its rubric the supposedly domestic and private scenes of family, school, church and trade union among others. Louis

ductive potency emerges in a phrase of Francis Bacon's quoted on the opening page of the first chapter of the book, "Concept of Enlightenment," and subsequently jumps the quotation marks to form a part of Adorno and Horkheimer's own text. Bacon deplores the vanities of uncritical dogmatic tradition as that which has hindered "the happy match between the mind of man and the nature of things."[4]

> … these and the like, have been the things which have forbidden the happy match between the mind of man and the nature of things; and in place thereof have married it to vain notions and blind experiments: and what the posterity and issue of so honourable a match may be, it is not hard to consider.[5]

Following Bacon's sarcasm with their own, Adorno and Horkheimer return to their own voices, wryly remarking that the marriage "is a patriarchal one: the mind, conquering superstition, is to rule over disenchanted nature." The thought of "disenchantment" offers a prelude to their basic position that the defeat of superstition transforms nature into abstract, domesticated matter even as it also enslaves the human understanding to its own disavowed nature (as domination). Relying on Henri Hubert and Marcel Mauss, their sources on "animism," Adorno and Horkheimer use mimeticism and incantation to provide the link in their argument, the correlation between knowledge and power, that will allow myth and enlightenment to flip in and out of each other's given terrain.

Whereas the sign, in myth, stood in community with things through their names, in enlightenment mastery, representation maintains the distance that facilitates a successful effort of control. In the first stage of the argument, the *likeness* between enlightenment and myth is drawn through their shared goal of mastery. Ritual performance attempts to intervene in natural process through mimetic invocation, while the urge to dominate actually succeeds in the scientific mastery of comprehended nature. Nonetheless, mimesis will turn up on the other side of the equation as an enduring trait of scientific operations as well. Adorno and Horkheimer execute this move – which may be considered the most important pivot point in their elaboration – to turn the logic of Freud's *Totem and Taboo* on its

---

Althusser, *Lenin and Philosophy and Other Essays*, trans. Ben Brewster (New York: Monthly Review Press, 2001), 85-126.

4 Francis Bacon, *Francis Bacon*, ed. Arthur Johnston (New York: Schocken Books, 1965), 15. Here is the translation from which Adorno and Horkheimer are working: … *dies und Ähnliches hat die glückliche Ehe des menschlichen Verstandes mit der Natur der Dinge verhindert, und ihn statt dessen an eitle Begriffe und planlose Experimente verkuppelt: die Frucht und Nachkommenschaft einer so rühmlichen Verbindung kann man sich leicht vorstellen.* (10)

5 Ibid.

head. With this turn, they open a new and complex historical relation between the mythic imagination and enlightenment reason, that is to say, they assert enlightenment's inability to recognize itself as the fullness of animist ambition.

> Die Zauberei ist wie die Wissenschaft auf Zwecke aus, aber sie verfolgt sie durch Mimesis, nicht in fortschreitender Distanz zum Objekt. Sie gründet keineswegs in der 'Allmacht der Gedanken', die der Primitive sich zuschreiben soll wie der Neurotiker; eine 'Überschätzung der seelischen Vorgänge gegen die Realität' kann es dort nicht geben, wo Gedanken und Realität nicht radikal geschieden sind. Die 'unerschütterliche Zuversicht auf die Möglichkeit der Weltbeherrschung', die Freud anachronistisch der Zauberei zuschreibt, entspricht erst der realitätsgerechten Weltbeherrschung mittels der gewiegteren Wissenschaft. (*DA*, 17)

> Magic like science is concerned with ends, but it pursues them through mimesis, not through an increasing distance from the object. It certainly is not founded on the "omnipotence of thought," which the primitive is supposed to impute to himself like the neurotic; there can be no "over-valuation of psychical acts" in relation to reality where thought and reality are not radically distinguished. The "unshakeable confidence in the possibility of controlling the world" which Freud anachronistically attributes to magic applies only to the more realistic form of world domination achieved by the greater astuteness of science. (*DE*, 7)

Here, Adorno and Horkheimer complicate the teleological schematization of Freud's "three great world-conceptions," and reveal an anachronism at the root of his historical inquiry, asserting that Freud's definition of animist belief instead corresponds to rampant industrialization. They diagnose their own project with the same stroke, however, since their basic understanding of mimetic ritual derives from the same scholarship cited in Freud's investigation. Here repetition takes on its most fatal power – as well as an ironic redoubling – as it moves through the dialectic until it successfully reproduces enlightenment as myth:

> Die Lehre der Gleichheit von Aktion und Reaktion behauptete die Macht der Wiederholung übers Dasein, lange nachdem die Menschen der Illusion sich entäußert hatten, durch Wiederholung mit dem wiederholten Dasein sich zu indentifizieren und so seiner Macht sich zu entziehen. Je weiter aber die magische Illusion entschwindet, um so unerbittlicher hält Wiederholung unter dem Titel Gesetzlichkeit den Menschen in jenem Kreislauf fest, durch dessen Vergegenständlichung im Naturgesetz er sich als freies Subjekt gesichert wähnt. Das Prinzip der Immanenz, der Erklärung jeden Geschehens als Wiederholung, das die Aufklärung wider die mythische Einbildungskraft vertritt, ist das des Mythos selber. Die trockene Weisheit, die nichts Neues unter der Sonne gelten läßt ... – diese trockene Weisheit reproduziert bloß die phantastische, die sie verwirft; die Sanktion des Schicksals, das durch Vergeltung unablässig wieder herstellt, was je schon war. (*DA*, 18)

> The doctrine that action equals reaction continued to maintain the power of repetition over existence long after humankind had shed the illusion that, by repetition, it could identify itself with repeated existence and so escape its power. But the more the illusion of magic vanishes, the more implacably repetition, in the guise of regularity, imprisons human beings in the cycle now objectified in the laws of nature, to which they believe they owe their security as free subjects. The principle of immanence, the explanation of every event as repetition, which enlightenment upholds against mythical imagination, is that of myth itself. The arid wisdom which acknowledges nothing new under the sun ... – this barren wisdom merely reproduces the fantastic doctrine it rejects: the sanction of fate which, through retribution, incessantly reinstates what always was. (*DE*, 8)

Though it is not possible to designate the alternation between the terms repetition and reproduction in the *Dialectic of Enlightenment* as a rigorous conceptual distinction, the passage above imparts some sense of their relation to one another. In the attempt to overcome the contagions of mimetic repetition, enlightenment gives itself over to an equally barren repetition that then bears a surprising fruit: the reproduction of mythology itself as enlightenment, a kind of alien birth.

One can observe a lingering organicist trace in Adorno and Horkheimer's jibe at Bacon in that they retain his ascription of barrenness to the dogmatic "marriage," on the one hand, and simultaneously disparage "reproduction" as secondary to production, on the other. Here they participate in an old Enlightenment legacy, a sense of threat posed by releasing the basic reproductivity of the imagination, in Kant's account, to its unexpectedly autonomous *productivity* in aesthetic judgments. As we know, aesthetic man will have to answer for the troubles of Enlightenment man. In the insinuation that enlightenment has been unable to parthenogenically *produce* itself without succumbing to a blind repetition – slipping from the autonomous to the automated – the simultaneous disavowal of reproduction as repetition and its guarding as the index of potency signals the continuance of an enlightenment problematic within Adorno and Horkheimer's critique.

Adorno and Horkheimer loosely define the goal of the enlightenment as "liberating humans beings from fear and setting them up as masters" (the first having been failed and the second all too well achieved) and Michel Foucault has offered the wonderful first definition of critique as "the art of not being governed quite so much."[6] For my own study, I would add to these definitions the project of emancipation that announces

---

6 Adorno and Horkheimer, *Dialectic of Enlightenment*, 1. German: Adorno and Horkheimer, *Dialektik der Aufklärung*, 9; Michel Foucault, *The Politics of Truth*, ed. Sylvère Lotringer (New York: Semiotext(e), 1997), 29.

itself in a corollary demand for collective equality, for that demand which both Ernst Bloch and Étienne Balibar have argued, in markedly variant interpretations of the *Déclarations* of 1789/93/95, to be liberty's corollary: equality.[7]

The impetus of the readings to follow thus derives from an interest in texts which attempt to assure a ground for equality in rational argumentation and still other texts which attend to the paradoxes of reason upon which these first texts, for all their attempt to do otherwise, founder. For nowhere is the failure of what is called enlightenment more apparent than in the concretization of human rights. In the paradoxical invocations of *habeas corpus* witnessed in the past two centuries both in the attempt to reapply rights to bodies alienated from sovereign spheres or in the attempt to restore enslaved bodies to a place before the law – whether within the disintegration of the institutions of American slavery or casual economies beyond any protection – the problem of fulfilling a body in natural law has posed a continual challenge.[8]

My study of what is called the Enlightenment through reference to the Age of Revolution in Europe is, no doubt, conditioned by the choice of texts I here read, texts which temporize with speculative histories, in the case of both the literary and the philosophical, and that participate in enlightenment while also attempting to supplement it. I choose these works, by Mary Shelley, Immanuel Kant, Johann Wolfgang von Goethe, Friedrich Schiller and Heinrich von Kleist, because they illumine one another's projects, and in them a central conundrum of "reproduction" still live in Adorno and Horkheimer's rhetoric takes a particular shape.

The "reproduction of enlightenment" entails questions of how precepts are passed down through generations, how subjects not vested with rights in their first declaration might "inherit" them and how enlightenment expands its territory through its presentation of the history of human knowledge production. Given the initial configuration of enlightenment liberation as one that still assumes inequality in the "domestic spheres" of labor, education, material sustenance and affective arrange-

---

7 See Ernst Bloch, *Naturrecht und menschliche Würde* (Frankfurt a.M.: Suhrkamp, 1961) [English: Ernst Bloch, *Natural Law and Human Dignity*, trans. Dennis J. Schmidt (Cambridge, Mass.: MIT Press, 1986)] and Étienne Balibar, *Masses, Classes, Ideas*, trans. James Swenson (New York: Routledge, 1994).

8 Here I am thinking of the paradoxical uses of *habeas corpus* (thou shalt have the body) in the Margaret Whittaker case upon which Toni Morrison drew for her novel *Beloved* and the current Supreme Court application of *habeas corpus* to gain some jurisdiction over the prison in Guantanamo Bay. In the case of casual economies in globalization, laboring bodies are also bereft of rights, because the *actual* international society of the economic has far outpaced any sphere of sovereignty that could plausibly assure them.

ments, these comparative readings scan for the representational strategies wherein a "body" becomes evident or legibile and then attempts to assimilate itself to the terms of "self-evidence" wherein its rights are named.

My readings thus begin with an appreciation of Shelley's epistolary novel, *Frankenstein: A Modern Prometheus*, as itself a reading of philosophical doubles conceived in the texts of three Enlightenment projects of liberation: Kant's *Critique of Practical Judgment*, Rousseau's *Discourse on the Origins of Inequality Among Men and Whether it is Justified by Natural Law*, and the *Declaration of the Rights of Man and the Citizen* (1793). In each of these texts a possibility for freedom is established through the conjuration of a double residing in the same mortal frame. In Shelley's epistolary novel, the abstractions deployed to depict these freedoms, particularly in the figure of self-evidence, are given over to a haunting of problems of reproduction. A liberated subject remains riven between the two modes of self-evidence: the rationally demonstrable on the one hand and the embodied, self-(re)producing, on the other.

The narrative logic of Shelley's novel exposes these philosophical "doubles" which respond to and negotiate contradictions between representation and reproduction. The doubles in question comprise instances of an apparent argumentative need to differentiate between the rational being and the human; natural pity and civilized man; man and the citizen, the individual and general will. Shelley's monster, most frequently called a "daemon," springs out of the universal designation on the other side of the human or man in each of these pairs. Though not man he might become a rational being possessed of natural pity, closer in character to the citizen and utterly subsumable under a general rubric. Further, the impossibility of conclusively identifying the novel's protagonist – the imbrications of autobiographical voices in its execution – points to the fiction at work in each of these philosophical doublings of the "same" and reveals it as an ethical dilemma: that of providing for a formal equality materially. Shelley's daemon demands a recognition that a formal equality cannot adequately address and exposes inequalities rooted in the disavowed social "facts" of reproduction – economic, cultural, material. In his partial access to these split categorical designations, either as rational being without being human or potential citizen without being man, Shelley's unlucky daemon also collapses the final pair general/individual in his community of one. Thus, his petition, eccentric to the project of human rights, but rather for the rights of the citizen *as a right to rights*, gestures emphatically toward the reproductive sphere as the scene of justice not accounted for in the formal equivalences of the law.[9] In this process, Shelley catches at the trick of reproduction as the negative index of the monster's peculiarly embodied claim, both in terms of the false grounds of universalism revealed by his being as part-protagonist but also in the curious narrative logic whereby he "embodies" a universal come to life.

Here my reading runs contrary to the habit of assessing Shelley's *Frankenstein* in the terms of technology critique or problems presented by the scientific penetration of the secrets of life (these would be much more consonant with critical responses to industrialization such as that offered in *Dialectic of Enlightenment* with its manifesto-like declarations *Technik ist das Wesen dieses Wissens*).[10] Though certainly it vividly characterizes both the scientific drive and the romantic genius run amok, Shelley's novel does not only emphasize the crisis of man striving to become god but even more so a series of paradoxes inherent to man becoming man. To this extent, it is not only important that the daemon represents an assemblage of reanimated dead-matter but also that he registers the becoming-living-matter of a generality.

Thus in the second chapter, we encounter Kant's definition of the natural organism (*Naturzweck*) in strictly formal terms as a self-(re)producing form which appears to human understanding to *set its own ends*. With this formal definition of the organism, Kant reintroduced the problem of entelechy to a materialist position whose radicalism up to that point had consisted in delimiting the investigation of nature to the divining of mechanistic (efficient) causes. In the second half of *Critique of Judgment*, the question arises as to whether the specifically human tendency to judge in terms of final causes might not present a heuristic for investigating living matter (living matter understood necessarily with respect to *living form*) in so far as organisms are witnessed to grow, heal, and reproduce themselves. Still, the teleological speculation undertaken in Kant's definition of the organism enters into a curious resonance with the larger project of *Critique of Judgment*, because matter that appears to be endowed, literally completely identical with a principle of living form, comes to constitute what Kant terms an "analogue of life" – a noteworthy move in that

9 For the context of Hannah Arendt's formulation of a 'right to rights' see "The Decline of the Nation-State and the End of the Rights of Man" in *The Origins of Totalitarianism* (Hannah Arendt, *The Origins of Totalitarianism* (New York: Harcourt, Brace and World, 1966). For a compelling contemporary discussion of Arendt's conception of "statelessness" see Judith Butler and Gayatri Chakravorty Spivak, *Who Sings the Nation State: Language, Politics, Belonging* (Calcutta: Seagull Books, 2007). See also Étienne Balibar, *Politics and the Other Scene*, trans. Christine Jones (New York: Verso, 2002).

10 Adorno and Horkheimer, *Dialektik der Aufklärung*, 10. "Technology is the essense of this knowledge. " (*DE*, 2).

"life" for Kant is principally defined as a desiring capacity, the ability to will.

The matter which comprises plants and animals in their growth doubles itself in that it also *appears to will* the form it becomes. Such an analogy will lead, in the farther reaches of the appendices of the third *Critique*, to the proposal of a further analogy between natural forms and the forms which undergird constitutional governance: the specific relation of the general to the particular. The judgment of living, material forms comes to encode for human understanding a paradoxical passage through the abyss between nature and freedom and to provide an image of itself: freedom comes into nature *as* human history. It is important in this passage, that the category of "human" thus announces itself as collectivity, and not as in the case of the ethics, the singular "reasoning being." [11]

Here again, though, the facilitiating figure of reproduction brings with it a certain risk, and my second chapter, "Generating Universals," circles back at its close to read organic metaphor in Kant's earlier, more popular writings on enlightenement and the possibility of a "universal" (*allgemein*) history. Between the two essays "Answer to the Question: What is Enlightenment?" and "Idea for a Universal History with a Cosmopolitan Purpose" reproduction figures human history as that of the growth of a seed to flourishing plant as well as the seemingly mechanized repetition of doctrine in religious communities and schools. Here the figure enables the possible engendering of history in nature but also a potential foreclosing of rational agency. Precisely that which could render human history writable and legible *in general* also threatens to annihilate it as closed, quantifiable system.[12] One runs up against something of a paradox of yet another order than that of the identity of freedom and necessity in *Critique of Practical Reason*: the living form, defined in terms of its reproduction, must overcome reproduction to produce itself as historical man. A dream not far from Dr. Frankenstein's. If we follow the identity of freedom and necessity (as demonstrated by reason alone) into the self-reflective terrain of aesthetic and teleological critique, the "abstract matter," which Adorno

11 On Kant's transformation of Rousseau's general will into an "idea" see Ernst Cassirer, *Rousseau, Kant, Goethe*, trans. James Gultman, Paul Oskar Kristeller & John Herman Randall, Jr. (Princeton: Princeton University Press, 1945).

12 In this sense, the fact that the essay begins with a reflection on rates of birth, death and marriage, brings Part Five of Foucault's *History of Sexuality* immediately to mind. Michel Foucault, *The History of Sexuality: An Introduction*, Vol. 1, trans. Robert Hurely (New York: Random House, 1978), 135-159. On the key issue of probability see Rudiger Campe's "Wahrscheinlich oder Scheinbar – mathematische Formel vs. philosophischer Diskurs (Quasi-Transzendental/Kant)" in *Spiel der Wahrscheinlichkeit: Literatur und Rechnung zwischen Pascal und Kleist* (Göttingen: Wallstein, 2002), 380-417.

and Horkheimer describe as the result of immanence-as-repetition, might *come to life* like Frankenstein's monster – but as the double of life, its "analogue."

In their generation of a positive concept of enlightenment Adorno and Horkheimer remark: "Causality was only the last philosophical concept on which scientific criticism tested its strength, because it alone of the old ideas still stood in the way of such criticism, the latest secular form of the creative principle." (*DE*, 3)[13] In Kant's *Critique of Judgment*, the judgment of an immanent causality, embedded in matter by new understandings of organic form, allows teleological judgment to speculate on purpose in human history. Not spirit, but rather the paradox of a simultaneously self-sufficient and *productive* will, a "natural purpose" (*Naturzweck*) that sets its own ends, brings about freedom in time. By reintroducing final causes as a heuristic in the observation of natural forms, Kant's "Critique of Teleological Judgment" offers one of the best glimpses of how the figure of organic form begins to root itself in understandings of culture.

The importance of an appropriable penchant toward freedom (that a nature of man could be appropriated to a history of freedom), while remaining largely suspended in Kant's critique, becomes more concrete in works following Kant's *Critique of Judgment* where it becomes a figure that allows for the legibility of history in cultural endeavors. The life-form, as more than mere mechanical repetition but also autopoeitic striving, comes to safeguard meaning where the previous suture between creator and its creature has begun to come undone. Shuttling between freedom (understood as willing self-determination) and nature (as the unswerving regularity of mechanical laws) without reaching an entirely stable point of transcendence, the richly productive grounds of cultural history begin to configure themselves. This non-transcendent life-form still points elsewhere, but also makes bodies self-indexing and retrieves the universal as the particular. A question still reverberates, though, from the unclosed frame of Kant's *Critique of Judgment*, if the universal returns as the immanent housed in living teleological forms, how does this new form condition subjects?

In distinct, but mutually resonant ways, the classical era stages of Goethe and Schiller take off from this problem. Goethe and Schiller's project for the Weimar classical stage understands the stage as a space that can reveal the body as an instance of the universal-as-particular. Conjuring

---

13 "Die Ursache war nur der letzte philosophische Begriff, an dem wissenschaftliche Kritik sich maß, gleichsam weil er allein von den alten Ideen ihr noch sich stellte, die späteste Säkularisierung des schaffenden Prinzips." (*DA*, 11)

with the artificiality of stage representation, Schiller articulates a program for a a new classical theater in his essay "On the Use of the Chorus" (written to accompany his tragedy *The Bride of Messina*) that proposes an imaginary distance between his audience and the figures on stage, a space that allows those figures neither to represent only themselves nor refer to some other determinate, though fictional, reality. Rather, Schiller's argument for a new theater elaborates a form of ideality that negotiates the estranged *reality* of the figure on stage in its "return" as a "generalized particular": the *natural* not as contingent but *ideal.* As Schiller puts it, the chorus destroys "everything that resists poetry" and saves the stage from mere mimesis. In this guise, the "natural" in Schiller's terms attains to the status of a simultaneously immediate and reflected form. Schiller's project for the stage thus attempts to give to perception an apprehension of the general in appearances. In this context, *life* takes on a distinctly cultural designation as the aesthetic embodiment of natural form shorn of its sheerly contingent status. The incestuous fatalities of Ancient Greek tragedy are returned to not as bourgeois tragedy but as a distanced ideal, *a mediated work of the imagination of the audience* which, protected by the wall of appearance set up by the chorus, perceives *itself* as much as it does the players on stage and what they enact.

For Goethe and Schiller both, the Weimar classical stage takes up questions of an elevated or mythic domestic sphere as the locus for the redemption of a sublimated politics.[14] For Schiller, the imaginatively distant but speaking presence of the body on stage compensates for the loss of political immediacy, and Goethe's treatment of the Iphigenia material in his play (*Schauspiel*) *Iphigenie auf Tauris* raises questions concerning violence and universal peace through a renewed staging of myth. Goethe's Iphigenia stands in a double position as the sister and daughter who can undo the crisis of patrilineal inheritance – free her brother from the curse of her mother in the name of her father. In so doing, however, she claims herself not to be speaking to her particular position as a member of the "Tantalus' Geschlecht" but to the general problem of the "Enlightenment of woman." In this mode, she renegotiates the problem of sacrifice at the

14 See Peter Hohendahl's discussion of Schiller's *Die Braut von Messina* in *Literary Paternity, Literary Friendship*, ed. Gerhard Richter (Chapel Hill: University of North Carolina, 2002). On the relation between Goethe's naturalist studies, his theater and his politics – "What reconciled poetry and politics in his eyes was not aesthetics, but the study of nature." – see Walter Benjamin's encyclcopedia article on Goethe in Walter Benjamin, *Gesammelte Schriften*, Bd. II.2 (Frankfurt a.M.: Suhrkamp, 1977), 705-739. Translated by Rodney Livingstone for *New Left Review* I/133, May-June, 1982.

heart of tragedy as the work of her own heart mirroring the will of the gods.[15]

Goethe's Iphigenie speaks from the *caesura* between her death forestalled and her life suspended. In her speech, she refigures the bloody sacrifice she was spared by viewing her new "life" as the mere tendance of her own grave, because she is bereft of family and fatherland. When Arkas asks her why she cannot be content in Tauris, she replies, "Kann uns zum Vaterland die Fremde werden?" (*Can to homeland the foreign accede?)* To which he responds, the two lines forming a chiasmus, "Und dir ist fremd das Vaterland geworden." (*And foreign did homeland become to you.)* Unlike the Marquise of O from Kleist's novella, Goethe's Iphigenie does not read her father's hand raised against her as rendering her alien.[16] Rather, she accepts the sacrifice as necessary and then attempts to generalize her own "second death" (life in Tauris) to the cause of universal peace. She thus internalizes the sacrifice once exterior to her and remythologizes her own story, not as that of entanglement in a fated house, but as the *universally human* as *woman*. The word *Geschlecht* in Goethe's play thus provides the crucial link between house of Tantalus and *Weiblichkeit*. Goethe plays provocatively here with some of the paradoxes that form Frankenstein's daemon's dilemma as the universal-as-singular, sexed subject.

If in different ways for both Goethe and Schiller, aesthetic *Anschauung* serves to access the universal *in* the particular, their variant comprehensions of the ideality of the natural alert us to a new possibility for figuring prospective historical fulfillment in a peculiarly aesthetic form of presence. In their collaborative letters on the distinction between epic and dramatic forms, the two authors insist upon the importance of the presence of the body on stage to achieve these theatrical effects. Arguing that the passional body enthralls the imagination of the audience, they insist that tragedy both generate and *transform* this reaction to a body on stage. In this sense, through a kind of binding or sacrifice, the classical stage allows the real to become the ideal by retaining and sublating this one moment of the real in embodied performance.

---

15 Thaos grimly notices the efficacy of her approach in an exchange attendant to her refusal of his unrefined proposal of marriage:

Thaos: Es spricht kein Gott; es spricht dein eignes Herz
Iphigenie: Sie reden nur durch unser Herz zu uns.

16 In Kleist's *Marquise of O*, when the Marquise's father reaches for his gun, she grabs her children and repairs to her summer estate. In so doing, she seems to figure paternal violence as a breach of the social contract and to assert her own sovereingty and paternity until she can successfully reinsert herself in the symbolic order through marriage to her assailant.

The significatory question of sacrifice so central to Goethe's *Iphigenie auf Tauris* remains important also for the denouement of Heinrich von Kleist's *Penthesilea, ein Trauerspiel.* For Goethe's play bloody sacrifice refers both to ancient sacral rites and the ill of xenophobia. It is the *bloody* sacrifice of the foreign that Iphigenie's presence in Tauris forestalls and which the general condition of her status *qua* woman is meant to undo through persuasive speech. In Kleist's *Trauerspiel*, in contrast, sacrifice does not form the locus of necessity but rather *comes into being* over the course of the tragic play. It is Penthesilea's execration that *turns into* sacrifice at play's end when Penthesilea drops the corpse of Achilles at the High Priestess' feet. Therefore, for Kleist's theater, ritual does not provide the prehistory or point of departure of the play's action but veritably becomes its product.

In his magnificent interpretation of Goethe's *Iphigenie auf Tauris*, Adorno offers a dialectical reading of the play that insists it not be reduced to a mere monument of classicism dedicated to a consolidation of the "human."[17] To argue this, Adorno notes that though Iphigenie implores Thaos to abandon his "barbaric custom, " it remains Thaos who has the power to (and does) grant this wish.[18] In this reversal of the logic of recognition and power, the "barbaric other" must incorporate and sustain the wish of civilization. This accomplished, the mythic repetition that has landed Iphigenie on Tauris' shores does not reproduce one more time but is instead transformed.

It is not difficult to note some trace of the myth/enlightenment dyad from *Dialectic of Enlightenment* in Adorno's reading. Adorno's dialectic saves Goethe from his own mythologization in the canons of German *Bildung* rather than trivialize him as the servant of one of enlightenment's most repeatable tropes: the intrinsic value of the "human."[19] The reading instead renders Goethe's text distinctly modern.[20] All the same, it is important to note that Iphigenie's plea for the universally human comes in the guise of her reference to her universalizable particularization as woman.

17 Theodor W. Adorno, *Notes to Literature*, vol. 2, trans. Shiery Weber Nicholson (New York: Columbia University Press, 1992), 153-170.

18 See also Peter Hohendahl discussion of Adorno's interpretation of *Iphigenie auf Tauris*. Peter Hohendahl, *Prismatic Thought* (Lincoln, University of Nebraska Press, 1997), 89-92.

19 As Adorno and Horkheimer put it: "Die Antwort des Ödipus auf das Rätsel der Sphinx: 'Es ist der Mensch' wird als stereotype Auskunft der Aufklärung unterschiedslos wiederholt ..." *Dialektik der Aufklärung*, 23. English: "Oedipus's answer to the riddle of the Sphinx – 'That being is man' – is repeated indiscriminately as enlightenment's stereotyped message...", 4.

20 "The historical-philosophical accent placed on the interaction between myth and the subject gives the text its unfading modern quality." Adorno, *Notes to Literature*, 155.

Further, despite the gradually accruing beauty of metaphors for listening and recognition over the course of the play, it presents its denouement with a kind of placidity that undermines any trace of transcultural risk.

In their treatment of sacrifice in "Concept of Enlightenment," Adorno and Horkheimer identify its semiotics as a way-station between what they call pantheism and discursive logic. This distinction derives principally from a theory of language which organizes the argument and owes much to Hegel, though Goethe's theory of the symbol may be as influential upon it. In this argument, the substitution at work in sacrifice takes us one step toward discursive logic: the goat, lamb, deer sacrificed already begin to represent *Gattung* (genre, species) but each also remains unique as the specifically chosen. Each remains "im Austausch unaustauschbar." The paradox of this formulation is reminiscent of a turn of phrase Goethe uses in a letter on the poetics of form:

> Kein Mensch will begreifen, daß die höchste und einzige Operation der Natur und Kunst die Gestaltung sei, und in der Gestalt die Spezifikation, damit jedes ein besonderes Bedeutendes werde, sei und bleibe.[21]
> Nobody wants to understand that the highest and only operation of nature and art is formation and in form [lies] the specification whereby everything becomes, is and remains a particular which also signifies.[22]

The curious eternity of this simultaneous becoming, abiding and being speaks directly to the resource Goethe will attribute to the symbol over against allegory. For the Goethe of this period, allegory transforms appearances into concepts, concepts into images, and then holds the concept stable, delimited, in the image. In contrast, the symbol changes appearances into ideas and ideas into images which then remain eternally active, just unreachable, at work in the image which both evades and consummates language's desire. The ideas in the symbolic image are "spoken" in all languages, but remain unspeakable. It may be the notion of such a "living concept" that informs Adorno and Horkheimer's renunciation of the very possibility in their thesis concerning the persistence of mythic repetition in the sureties of discursive logic.

> Die Lehre der Priester war symbolisch in dem Sinn, daß in ihr Zeichen und Bild zusammenfielen. Wie die Hieroglyphen bezeugen, hat das Wort ursprünglich auch die Funktion des Bildes erfüllt. Sie ist auf die Mythen übergegangen. Mythen wie magische Riten meinen die sich wiederholende Natur. Sie ist der Kern des Symbolischen: ein Sein oder ein Vorgang, der als ewig vorgestellt wird, weil er im Vollzug des Symbols stets wieder Ereignis wer-

21 Cited in Sørensen, Bengt Algot: "Die 'zarte Differenz'" in *Formen und Funktionen der Allegorie,* hrsg. Walter Haug (Stuttgart : J.B. Metzlersche, 1979) 640.

22 Reese translation.

> den soll. Unerschöpflichkeit, endlose Erneuerung, Permanenz des Bedeuteten sind nicht nur Attribute aller Symbole, sondern ihr eigentlicher Gehalt. (23)

> The teachings of the priests were symbolic in the sense that in them sign and image coincided. As the hieroglyphs attest, the word originally also had a pictorial function. This function was transferred to myths. They, like magic rites, refer to the repetitive cycle of nature. Nature as self-repetition is the core of the symbolic: an entity or a process which is conceived as eternal because it is reenacted again and again in the guise of the symbol. Inexhaustibility, endless renewal, and the permanence of what they signify are not only attributes of all symbols but their true content. (12)

The complexity of both Schiller's understanding of the modern instantiation of the chorus and Goethe's presentation of dramatic speech can remind us of the kind of remythologization of nature pointed to in the work of Adorno and Horkheimer, but *not* just as mechanized repetition or the leveling equivalence of abstract universalization, but *also* an emergent alignment of human cognition with natural form – an allegory that must be forgotten in order to function. The life-form stabilizes the becoming meaningful of *beings* partly by approximating them to living signs. The quicksand of this paradox begins to dissolve the historical content of Goethe's play even though Iphigenie manages to talk her way out of myth and into history, a process cast as the overcoming of ritual repetition. Goethe's *Iphigenie* thus stages the emergence of tragedy itself as the dialogue with and distanciation from its own ("barbaric") precedents – as a defeat of reproduction in favor of historical singularity. Goethe's "Schauspiel" overcomes the tragic logic – the inevitability of mythic repetition – that Adorno and Horkheimer ascribe to the real history of western civilization to such an extent that it can no longer register as tragedy.

Iphigenie's suspended sacrifice allows her to move in a ground beyond the contingent. In this way, her own description of the form of her speech in Goethe's play points to a kind of irreplaceable immediacy that nonetheless houses the generality of her claims for *die Aufklärung des Weibes* (the Enlightenment of woman). Paradoxically, her actions should actually resolve the dilemma that first grounds her speech in the double space of her sublated sacrifice. She works to bring an end to the repetition of ritual, but the conditions of her campaign rely on the *reproduction* of her other, in Thoas, as the limit of history: an infinitely repeatable procedure that carries on through Adorno and Horkheimer's very designation of "animism" as the limit towards which enlightenment itself designates its own fall.

* * *

Kleist's *Penthesilea: Ein Trauerspiel* revisits the logic whereby one's foreign interloctur comes to designate the limit or threshold of history. His fantasmatic fictional myth of Penthesilea, leader of the Amazons, though drawing obliquely on classical sources announces itself as specifically fictive and new – especially in that its denouement undoes the ending of Homer's *Iliad*, leaving the outcome of the Trojan war in question and the Greeks bereft of Achilles. Most importantly, Kleist's tragic drama actively eschews any safe transit between particular and universal but rather presents such a possibility as a dynamic site of risky and *contingent* passage, wherein even the repetition of a name can become a mistranslation.

Whereas Goethe and Schiller contrast the freedom granted the imagination by the invisible voice of the rhapsodist to the binding immediacy of the actor's body, Kleist merges the two to produce what might be called a concretized epic poetics of the stage. Kleist's *Trauerspiel stages* epic utterances, producing unpredictable theatrical effects, and destablizing the certainties of embodied vision. Far from the living eternity of the symbol, Kleist's stage poetics are more aptly described by the terms Walter Benjamin used to designate Baroque allegory: "Any person, any object, any relationship can mean absolutely anything else."[23] Thus Achilles' male body visible on stage is described to the spectator's imagination as a "slender necked doe" while the staggering strength and speed of Penthesilea's movement off stage is strained after with a constantly shifting series of epic similes: she gusts like a hurricane wind, tossing Greek soldiers before her, winds like a snake out of the mountains, seeks her query with the hunger and speed of a wolf running across snow. Penthesilea has been so lengthtily and impossibly described before her appearance on stage that the actor's body must come forth more as a riddle when once it appears. And yet the doubling that takes place here cannot be described as that between essence and appearance, force and effect. Penthesilea registers an effect without knowable or locatable force, an appearance without an essence. The idea that language evolves through the invocation of the spirit indwelling in any particular being or thing contrasts with Kleist's theater to the extent that every thing and being seems to provide a fugitive site of passage for a force that moves through phenomena, relating them not to themselves in abstraction, but to other things, or at least, through dint of the abstractions they come to house or bear, they also fall into and out of relation with other things *and* words through sheer contiguity.

If the order of representation remains crucial for Adorno and Horkheimer's dialectic, it does so on the basis of mimesis understood as the

---

23 Benjamin, Walter. *The Origin of German Tragic Drama*, trans. John Osbourne (London: NLB, 1977), 175.

legacy of preanimist thinking in the logical equivalences of discursive logic. To serve this purpose, mimesis must be regarded as having a lost religious content that prefigures universalizing abstractions and actively forges the history of the conceptual itself.

> Die Verdoppelung der Natur in Schein und Wesen, Wirkung und Kraft, die den Mythos sowohl wie die Wissenschaft erst möglich macht; stammt aus der Angst der Menschen, deren Ausdruck zur Erklärung wird … Die Spaltung von Belebtem und Unbelebtem, die Besetzung bestimmter Orte mit Dämonen und Gottheiten, entspringt erst aus diesem Präanimismus. In ihm ist selbst die Trennung von Subjekt und Objekt schon angelegt. Wenn der Baum nicht mehr bloß als Baum sondern als Zeugnis für ein anderes, als Sitz des Mana angesprochen wird, drückt die Sprache den Widerspruch aus, daß nämlich etwas es selber und zugleich etwas anderes als es selber sei, identisch und nicht identisch. Durch die Gottheit wird die Sprache aus der Tautologie zur Sprache. Der Begriff, den man gern als Merkmalseinheit des darunter Befaßten definiert, war vielmehr seit Beginn das Produkt dialektischen Denkens, worin jedes stets nur ist, was es ist, indem es zu dem wird, was es nicht ist. (*DA*, 21)

> The doubling of nature into appearance and essence, effect and force, made possible by myth no less than science, springs from human fear, the expression of which becomes its explanation. … The split between animate and inanimate, the assigning of demons and deities to certain specific places, arises from this preanimism. Even the division of subject and object is prefigured in it. If the tree is adressed no longer as simply a tree but as evidence of something else, a location of *mana*, language expresss the contradiction that it is at the same time itself and something other than itself, identical and not identical. Through the deity speech is transformed from tautology into language. The concept, usually defined as the unity of the features of what it subsumes, was rather, from the first, a product of dialectical thinking, in which each thing is what it is only by becoming what it is not. (*DE*, 10-11)

Kleist's theater complicates this schema in that it reveals the ideal not hovering within but somehow *beside* the real. This space-beside parallels the peculiar space of Kleist's stage which does not remain constant as the self-same but is literally occupied (*besetzt*) by warring orders of representation. The space-beside as the stage itself assures that contiguity becomes more important than correlation in the lightening speed of the play of meaning. Even the proper name is mobile in Kleist, as the attempt to capture and recapture Penthesilea's name, and what this name signifies at any given moment, increasingly absorbs the action of the play. Ultimately, the very repetition of her name from different mouths collapses it into the "Musik der Rede" as which Penthesilea correctly understood Achilles had taken her words. Words are thus not only exchanged in Kleist's tragic play but are also exchanged as things, as sensual objects and impenetrable riddles.

Notably, one of the first conundra concerning Penthesilea is voiced by Antilochus (a name which could read as *anti-place*) in the first scene.

> Antilochus. Und niemand kann, was sie uns will, ergründen?
> Diomedes. Kein Mensch, das eben ist's … (1.162-63)[24]

> Antilochus: And none can fathom what she wants from us?
> Diomedes: That's just it, no one knows ... [25]

The first criterion of Penthesilea's inscrutability remains the inability of the Greeks to fathom (ground) her desire. At the level of the play's content, we could say that Penthesilea refuses the demand to be identical to her wishes or subsumable to the self-identity of her will. Thus she strays far from the logic of the *Naturzweck* of Kant's formal description. Bearing rather an assemblage of particular traits and tokens that neither resolve into a whole nor remain identical in time, Penthesilea's inscrutability presents a retreat from self-determination as the predominant mode for establishing truth. Here invocation, adjective and substantive blend into a play of forces that speak through being non-identical, by revealing the transfers of language in their movements. Where the tragic subject must stand on one ground but inhabit two, Penthesilea remains in constant motion and the universals which would hope to subsume her instance only race in a half-light behind. Nonetheless, Penthesilea is fatally stopped by play's end. In inverse directon to Goethe's Iphigenie, she speaks herself back into myth, into the death of her lover whose signature crime she has duplicated. Achilles' attempt to decode her desire through the codification of custom leads him to mistake her ultimate single act of combat (historically singular action) as a signifying ritual (repetition of myth). Thinking he can empty out sacrifice as a play, mere gesture, he enters the field unarmed. Penthesilea has meanwhile understood his use of metaphor to be a subterfuge and collapses all distance between image, sign and act. Through this paradox she either alienates her own consciousness or unexpectedly *generates* ritual out of historical time.

Penthesilea cannot be transposed into the "the Enlightenment of woman." Where Frankenstein's daemon has need of "reproduction" and demands it of enlightenment values which fail to recognize him, Penthesilea cannot escape reproduction *as translation* – the transposition of every

---

24 Heinrich von Kleist, *Sämtliche Werke und Briefe*, vol. 2, ed. Hans Rudolf Barth et al. (Frankfurt am Main: Deutscher Klassiker Verlag, 1987), 143-256.

25 Heinrich von Kleist, *Penthesilea: A Tragic Drama*, trans. Joel Agee (New York: Harper Collins Publishers, 1998), 9.

name through its repetition not in monolgue but in a dialogue that moves too fast. A fellow traveler with Thaos, she cannot lay the ground of recognition from which history will spring but she can return the ethical, dialogic and radically morphic dimension to a language otherwise content to resolve in self-evidence.

The positive concept Adorno and Horkheimer claim for enlightenment calls for a revitalization of the "theoretical imagination." In the readings which follow, I trace a series of figures of self-determination which in their imagining both rely upon and negate their own reproducibility, an aspect of their generation that bears the inextinguishable trace of social, embodied being. In so doing, this book hopes to discover the mobility of imaginations that seek the challenge of justice beyond commensuration.

Chapter One

Another Reasoning Being

> Hence the distinction between things possible and actual is such that it holds merely subjectively, for human understanding. For even if something does not exist, we can still have it in our thoughts; or we can present something as given, even though we have as yet no concept of it.
> – Immanuel Kant, *Critique of Judgment*

> As I said this I suddenly beheld the figure of a man, at some distance, advancing towards me with superhuman speed. He bounded over the crevices in the ice among which I had walked with caution …
> – Mary Shelley, *Frankenstein*

Since it first appeared in 1818, Mary Shelley's *Frankenstein* has been variously regarded as a repudiation of Enlightenment projects for political liberation, an incendiary extension of them or as the record of a vexed ambivalence with respect to notions of progress in general.[1] Having long

---

1 Portions of this chapter appeared in *Representations* 96 (Fall 2006), 48-72. The novel possesses a singular capacity to take on meaning and spark the imagination. Its unnamed monster comes forward with so shadowy an existence that he has been able to catalyze paradigmatic readings in numerous, often conflicting, methodologies. These include biographical, narratological, feminist, psychoanalytic, deconstructive, postcolonial, history of science, and technology studies approaches to the reading of texts. The scholarship is too vast to synthesize in one footnote, though I will touch on a number of seminal works of criticism which reflect these methods of reading. For an extremely helpful introduction to the scholarship of the "Frankenstein industry" see Berthold Schoene-Harwood, ed., *Mary Shelley: Frankenstein* (New York: Columbia University Press, 2000). James O'Rourke gives a summary of the reception history of the novel in terms of Enlightenment texts and the French Revolution before launching his own extremely thorough account of Mary Shelley's reading of Jean-Jacques Rousseau. James O'Rourke "'Nothing More Unnatural': Mary Shelley's Revision of Rousseau," *ELH* 56 (1989): 543-69. See also Lee Sterrenburg, "Mary Shelley's Monster: Politics and Psyche in *Frankenstein*," in *The Endurance of Frankenstein*, ed. George Levine and U.C. Knoepflmacher (Berkeley: University of California Press, 1979) 143-71; Fred Botting, "Reflections of Excess: *Frankenstein*, the French Revolution and Monstrosity," in *Reflections of Revolution: Images of Romanticism*, ed. Alison Yarrington and Kelvin Everest (London and New York: Routledge, 1993), 26-38; Chris Baldick, "The Politics of Monstrosity," in *New Casebooks: Frankenstein*, ed. Fred Botting (New York: Macmil-

since passed into the status of modern myth, the novel becomes uncannily evocative, not only through its imagining of the reanimation of lifeless matter, but also through its tripping of a series of paradoxes inherent to arguments on natural rights in the 18th century. Neither an endorsement nor rejection of the Enlightenment, the novel reveals a critical dilemma for attributions of the human proceeding from enlightenment.

In Kant's ethics, in Rousseau's politics, and in the *Declaration of the Rights of Man and the Citizen* (1789/1793) the identity of the "human" is split. *Frankenstein*'s staging of the non-humanness of Shelley's unnamed daemon contrasts with the split in the fundamental category of the "human" to be observed in this series of pivotal philosophical and political "doubles." The monster's peculiar relationship to acceding to a social form of existence thus brings to light an impasse faced by political subjects in 18th-century philosophy and allows for a new reading of them. Shelley's monster, that "figure of a man," moves across the shifting terrain of his own indetermination at "superhuman speed" (362); traversing the slash between man/citizen, reasoner/human, general/individual will in ways that pose a delicate challenge to the work of reason in enlightenment projects for a new authorization of law.[2]

Frankenstein presents the coming-into-being and embodiment of its daemon as a narrative challenge. The production and animation of the monster make up both the content and the *formal principle* of the narrative. In her retrospective "Author's Introduction" to the 1831 edition of *Frankenstein*, Shelley draws a sharp distinction between "the radiance of brilliant imagery" and the "machinery of a story." Emphasizing the cathexis not of a single image but of a *succession* of them, she identifies concatenation as the significant factor in the form.[3] Narrating the appearance of the vision

---

lan, 1995), 48-67. On Enlightenment and monstrosity see Barbara Maria Stafford, *Body Criticism: Imaging the Unseen in Enlightenment Art and Medicine* (Cambridge: MIT Press, 1991), 256-66.

2 Mary Shelley, *Frankenstein; or, The Modern Prometheus*, in *Three Gothic Novels*, ed. Peter Fairclough (New York: Penguin, 1988), 261. For convenience's sake, I will cite the 1831 version from the Penguin edition rather than from the footnoted variants at the end of the Pickering edition. Citations of the 1818 edition in brackets refer to Mary Shelley, *Frankenstein, or the Modern Prometheus*, vol. 1 of *The Novels and Selected Works of Mary Shelley*, ed. Nora Crook and Pamela Clemit (London: W. Pickering, 1996).

3 Schoene-Harwood writes that Shelley's 1831 introduction ultimately effects "a deplorable diffusion of *Frankenstein's* profoundly political impact and significance"; Schoene-Harwood, *Mary Shelley: Frankenstein*, 16. I will read the "following of trains of thought" instead as offering the crux of the novel's political engagement. See also James P. Carson, "Bringing the Author Forward: *Frankenstein* through Mary Shelley's Letters," *Criticism* 30 (1988): 431-53; Mary Poovey, "My Hideous Progeny: Mary Shelley and the Feminization of Romanticism," *PMLA* 95 (1980): 332-47; and Bette London, "Mary Shelley, *Frankenstein* and the Spectacle

at the center of her story, Shelley recapitulates the principle incidents of the first half of the novel, stopping at the point at which "the hideous phantasm of a man" opens the curtain and looks at his maker with "yellow, watery, but speculative eyes." Later, the process of his assemblage and animation are depicted as forming an inexorable chain of events that culminates in the dramatic encounter of monster and maker, a scene which increasingly consumes the novel's plot and has its first reprise in the speech on Mont Blanc in which the daemon declares "his right" to the society of a companion, indeed to society itself. A crisis of succession thus forms the dramatic core of the novel: autonomy succeeds upon production and paradoxically sets a relentless mechanism of plot into motion, leading ultimately to the crisis of a disputed inheritance. The non-human monster seeks to inherit the rights of man and the citizen from his progenitor.

Versions of a Sister *or* The Monster's Antecedents

Critics have generally agreed that the revisions of the Standard 1831 edition of Mary Shelley's novel *Frankenstein* served to tone the original 1818 edition down a bit.[4] In contrast to the anonymously authored original

of Masculinity," *PMLA* 108 (1993): 253-67. Fred Botting notes that Shelley's reference to a "waking-dream" has also reinforced the temptation to read the novel symptomatically; Fred Botting, *Making Monstrous: Frankenstein, Criticism, Theory* (Manchester: Manchester University Press, 1991), 80.

4 As Paul O'Flinn has argued, the later version can be said to reflect the emendations of a "more conservative and religious Mary Shelley ... so that we find her insisting in the 1831 introduction: 'supremely frightful would be the effect of any human endeavor to mock the stupendous mechanism of the Creator of the world.' She herself, in fact, is among the first to nudge the text into the space occupied by the determinant ideology, and we can also see that nudging going on in some of the revisions she makes for this third 1831 edition; for example, Elizabeth Lavenza is no longer Frankenstein's cousin, so that the potentially offensive hint of incest is deleted, while the orthodox notion of the family as moral and emotional sanctuary is boosted by the addition of several passages in the early chapters idealizing the domestic harmony of Frankenstein's childhood." In his reading of the ideological usages of Shelley's novel, O'Flinn proposes that these changes reflect Mary Shelley's proposal for one such use. Paul O'Flinn, "Production and Reproduction: The Case of *Frankenstein*," in *The Study of Popular Fiction*, ed. Bob Ashley (London: Pinter Publishers, 1989), 23-39. For an in-depth discussion of the differences between the various extant manuscripts of the novel see a series of essays by David Ketterer: "The Corrected *Frankenstein*: Twelve Preferred Readings in the Last Draft," *English Language Notes* 33, no. 1 (Sept. 1995), 23-35, and "(De) Composing *Frankenstein*: The Import of Altered Character Names in the Last Draft," *Studies in Bibliography: Papers of the Bibliographical Society of the University of Virginia* 49 (1996): 232-276.

edition, the revisions elide the implication of incest between Victor Frankenstein and Elizabeth Lavenza. Further, the "Author's Introduction" of 1831 offers a muted version of literary invention, attributing it to involuntary, dream visions instead of active production. I would like to revisit both these revisions. In the first case, Elizabeth changes from Frankenstein's cousin to a non-blood relation of a kind "no expression can body forth." In the second, Shelley's description of the novel's provenance as a "waking dream" importantly contrasts different modes of "embodying" ideas in literary form. In both instances the power of words and images to impart "body" as well as the name for a particular kind of "relation," whether it be social, as between persons, or cognitive, as between ideas and their "shape," is at stake.

Let us consider the first change. After shifting the circumstances so that Elizabeth is no longer Frankenstein's cousin, the first chapter of the Doctor's narrative closes:

> All praises bestowed on her I received as made to a possession of my own. We called each other familiarly by the name of cousin. No word, no expression could body forth the kind of relation in which she stood to me – my more than sister, since till death she was to be mine only. (Penguin 294)

Doctor Frankenstein strains to find an expression appropriate to the manifold aspects of his relation to Elizabeth that comprehend adopted sister, childhood playmate, and bride-to-be through early arrangement. In contrast, the 1818 edition offers an extended passage with a vivid description of Elizabeth:

> Her person was the image of her mind; her hazel eyes, although as lively as a little bird's, possessed an attractive softness. Her figure was light and airy; and, though capable of enduring great fatigue, she appeared the most fragile creature in the world. While I admired her understanding and fancy, I loved to tend on her, as I should on a favourite animal; and I never saw so much grace both of person and mind united to so little pretension. (23)

This passage, excised in 1831, offers to "body" Elizabeth – as animal, bird or insect – and to trace parallels between her "person" and her mind. The later version, on the other hand, abandons metaphor for variable-like, algebraic locutions such as "more than sister" and "kind of relation." While there are considerable grounds for regarding many of Shelley's later revisions of the novel as intended to emphasize the moral prescription of the tale and to impart Victorian values to the presentation of Franken-

---

Though arguments in favor of using the 1818 edition often bear witness to the social oppressions of Shelley's later life, they also have the unfortunate effect of discrediting the author's final editorial emendations.

stein's family, I note that this revision – though rendering Elizabeth Victor's cousin only *in name* – also introduces a blank space, a failure to name, to designate a determinate *relation*. The revision introduces a zone of signification as yet impossible to fill. The change may do more than exclude the possibility of incest; it may also conjure alternate possibilities.

The later version extends the entire section concerning Elizabeth's adoption in which the complicated series of non-original relations to which she is heir is played out. She modulates from being the daughter of Frankenstein's paternal aunt, to emerging amid her first adoptive family of peasants as in a fairy tale and "as of a distinct species." The orphaned "daughter of a Milanese nobleman" in the later edition, Elizabeth undergoes two adoptions before becoming Frankenstein's "more than sister" in 1831. The incestuous implication thus reverberates through two removes (just as the monster's narration of his life will echo through two frames). Offered the orphaned girl as a "present," the young Victor interprets the words literally and intercepts Elizabeth's praises, conceiving of her as the almost-proper, the nearly self-same. Notably, the question of *property* introduces the interruptive category or catechristic measure of intimacy against which the Doctor's enunciation attempts to present itself. The indirection of the phrase "all praises bestowed on her I received as made to a possession of my own" replaces the comparison drawn between Elizabeth and a favorite animal. (294) Her indeterminate category thus wavers in and out of the various possible approaches to naming the domestic relation of the would-be marriage: property, procreative capital, domestic servant, companion or pet. In one sense, Elizabeth's relation to Victor is complicated by her adoptive presence in Frankenstein's family, but the problem of naming her social status in terms of property was common to woman-in-marriage in general for the period.[5] The 1831 edition actually works to render this difficulty more abstract.

Elizabeth's close connection to Frankenstein is dislodged, however, by the appearance and coming-into-being of the other body that fills the multiple frames of the novel: that of the monster. From his figure, the motive force of the plot takes its impetus even as his increasingly panoptical presence endlessly retards the forward motion of the conventional

5 For an introductory and philosophically informed discussion of debates on marriage in the period see Carol Pateman, *The Sexual Contract* (Cambridge: Polity, 1988). A perusal of Mary Wollstonecraft's novel *Maria: Or the Wrongs of Woman* imparts a vivid sense of the situation. Mary Shelley's journals record that she was reading Wollstonecraft's *A Vindication of the Rights of Woman* alongside Locke in one period of *Frankenstein*'s composition. For readings on the history of marriage in modern Europe see also Richard Wall, Tamara K. Jareven, and Joseph Ehmer, ed., *Family History Revisited: Comparative Perspectives* (Newark: University of Delaware Press, 2001).

marriage plot never brought to achievement in Shelley's novel. The monster, slave, being, creature, or daemon possesses a similarly difficult-to-figure proximity to the Doctor who produced him. Seen as a "figure of a man," he might potentially share in the full range of abstract alternative appellations: such as reasoning being, citizen, or person.[6] What impairs his access to these forms of recognition, however, is precisely his particular form of embodiment and his self-proclaimed dependency on the man who produced him. He thus can be argued to more closely resemble the individuals who make up the unacknowledged "private sphere" of much political and social thought in the eighteenth century: women, slaves, and servants. I would suggest, then, that the blank space left between a body, a social relation, and a name for Frankenstein's "more than sister," in the 1831 edition does more than erase the implication of incest. It points to the insufficiency of the categories of relation that the monster's very existence, as we shall see, will more radically demonstrate than does Elizabeth's, that "apparition of a child."[7] The altered approach toward description also puts forth a principle of literary formation. With this move, the novel sets up a variable of correlation that becomes a *factor* for the rest of the novel. How are we to name social relations and what kinds of bodies do these names "body forth"?

The Figure of a Man

The question of the monster's status provides the thrice repeated impetus of the novel. First, his fleeting appearance in the arctic waste forms the "accident" of Walton's exploration; second, the possibility of his formation and animation drives Frankenstein's fate along "insensible steps" up to the moment of the daemon's animation; and finally, the daemon himself narrates the course of his development up to the point before which he appears in order to make his demand. Once this demand for a female

6 Shelley, *Frankenstein,* 362.

7 The vast body of criticism produced on Shelley's novel in the last thirty years testifies to the incredible proliferation of associative networks that the crafting and wording of this novel can sustain. Here already the language of the "apparition" haunts the first "vision" of Elizabeth as the object of Victor's father's gaze. Physical and psychic effects already mix in the registers of the word choice. As is the case when Walton desires an interlocutor and the Arctic landscape conjures him one, here Frankenstein's mother is miraculously provided with the daughter she had "much desired." The chain of incidents leading to the appearance of a new, apparently unmothered body is, however, in this instance, that of adoption as opposed to manual production (*Novels and Selected Works of Mary Shelley*, vol. 1, 192). In this sense, the arbitrary but "necessary" series of narrative incidents in Shelley's novel anticipate later science fiction concerns with the trap of materially manifested psychic desires such as the ocean in Stanislaw Lem's *Solaris* (Krakow: Wydawn. Literackie, 1994).

companion has been made, the novel proceeds to play out a fierce series of apparently unavoidable consequences. Victor Frankenstein's project to produce "life" leads directly to a proliferation of "mechanisms," and the novel abounds with unchecked and uncontrollable machination. Even Walton intuits something incomprehensible "working" in his soul before meeting Dr. Frankenstein, who himself describes his own being as a "mechanism." In describing his fatal attendance of lectures in *Naturphilosophie* in Germany, he relates:

> Such were the professor's words – rather let me say such the words of the fate – enounced to destroy me. As he went on I felt as if my soul were grappling with a palpable enemy; one by one the various keys were touched which formed the *mechanism* of my being; chord after chord was sounded, and soon my mind was filled with one thought, one conception, one purpose. (Penguin 307-8)

The Doctor's quest transforms him into an instrument (by all appearances an organ), or immutable drive, activated by Professor Waldman's enunciation. Notably, the importance of mechanism both precedes and issues from the production of the daemon here. After the Doctor is driven by a "resistless" urge to perform the experiment, the success of further experiment releases the daemon into action. The monster then comes to move the plot in keeping with the monotonous aims of the Doctor's drives. Like the *daemon* of fate so frequently invoked by Sophocles' Oedipus, the monster proceeds to stalk his creator *from ahead*. Dr. Frankenstein is forced to recognize his fate in the work of his own hand, or rather, in what that first work, now alien, continues to effect. Meanwhile, the daemon's autonomy is compromised in that it comes to describe a shadow history of the Doctor's "machinic" psyche. Questions of autonomy and automation[8] become inextricably linked as the identity of daemon and Doctor fuse and subdivide within the exigencies of the plot structure. Leaving a trail of destruction in his wake that looks like the negative image

---

8 For a reading of the novel's relation not to evolutionary theory but to technology see Mark Hansen, "Parody of Romantic Poetics in *Frankenstein*," in *SiR* 36 (Winter 1997): 575-609. Hansen argues, among other things, that Shelley contravenes enlightenment philosophers such as Condillac, Diderot, and "especially Rousseau" by locating a split not between nature/culture but "*within* culture (or, more precisely, *within* technology itself) ... " (584). Hansen is alert to the ways in which "Shelley's fictional monster functions 'machinically,' to appropriate Deleuze-Guattari's term, forging connections which *exceed* textual strategies of legitimation. Insofar as it 'gives birth' to something it cannot contain, *Frankenstein* performs the very techno-logic it explores, and in so doing, comes to function as a reality-check on the logocentrism of romantic poets" (580).

of the Doctor's desire, the daemon's animation seems to mechanize the Doctor's soul while simultaneously re-embodying it.[9]

When considering the structure of the narrative of Shelley's novel *Frankenstein,* the monster's peculiar body and process of coming into embodiment can be related structurally to the question of the protagonist, for who is the protagonist of the tale half-framed by Walton's letters: the Doctor or the manufactured man? One might confront the dilemma by sorting protagonists by frame, and calling the daemon the protagonist of the inner or ultimate narrative, in which he chronicles his own existence. This story, however, "ends" in the dramatic dialogue that takes place on Mont Blanc between the two leading figures of the previously distinct but entangled narratives. At this point, the monster's oral history folds out into the overarching narrative, which had begun by framing it.[10] He passes from his own self-narration into the second-level tale of Dr. Frankenstein's progress. It is here that he voices the demand that he be produced a companion, and the two sides of the mask now confront each other as in a drama. Meanwhile, the *thought* of the produced being had already long dominated the level of the narrative "proper" to Dr. Frankenstein – the monster is present prior to his "creation" as a *Trieb* or mania – but when he comes into being, he further freights the narrative with a haunting possibility, a demanded but not actualized future existence. Speaking in Viktor Shklovsky's terms, one could regard this as a framing device whereby one mask of the narrator is exchanged for another in order to

---

9 This aspect of the novel has rendered it remarkably germane to psychoanalytic construction. For two sustained analyses of the myriad possibilities introduced by such an approach to reading *Frankenstein* see Botting, *Making Monstrous.* Also Paul Sherwin, "*Frankenstein*: Creation as Catastrophe," *PMLA* 96 (1981): 883-903.

Dr. Frankenstein insists that his early experiments were methodical and within the realm of possibility: "Some miracle might have produced it, yet the stages of the discovery were distinct and probable," he says (36). Nonetheless, the "painful labor" and "gratifying consummation" of his toils immediately produce an uncontrollable psychic response. His work's consummation erases the history of the progress that performed it. The doctor continues: "this discovery was so great and overwhelming that all the steps by which I had been progressively led to it were obliterated, and I beheld only the result" (36). Similarly, the first recognition of the daemon's criminal activity comes in this vein: "The mere presence of the idea was irresistible proof of the fact" (55).

10 To invoke Beth Newman's reading, the letters that compose the multiple narratives reverse the usual relationship between text and voice in the period: "In this respect, *Frankenstein*, with its roots in the novels and romances of the previous century, takes a hackneyed convention and turns it nearly inside out. Instead of an editor producing a (supposedly) found manuscript, an already written document, Walton turns oral narratives into writing" Beth Newman, "The Frame Structure of *Frankenstein*," in *New Casebooks: Frankenstein*, ed. Fred Botting (London: MacMillan Press, 1995), 170.

connect a number of tales.[11] As Barbara Johnson has noted, the novel "presents not one but three autobiographies of men,"[12] although Beth Newman points out, on the other hand, that all three involve remarkable similarities of tone, word choice, and textual voice. One "autobiography" cedes to the next up to the point at which two masks meet in what could also be taken for an encapsulated closet drama at the core of the novel's structure: the monster's requisition or declaration.

In her own narrative construction of the logic of an origin within this almost machinic impetus of the plot, Shelley plays on the role of origin stories in Enlightenment treatments of natural law. Though childhood had already been invented by the time *Frankenstein* appeared, the monster notably lacks one. His "upbringing" instead reads like a variation on eighteenth-century "philosophical fictions." In his recitation of his life, he charts his cognitive progress moving, in Lockean vein, from pure unsorted sense perception, to the formation of ideas, and eventually to the attainment of literacy.[13] This trajectory closely resembles various mid-century speculations on the early development of spoken and written

---

11 Viktor Shlovsky, *Theory of Prose*, trans. Benjamin Sher (Elmwood Park, Ill.: Dalkey Archive Press, 1990). See chapter 3, "The Structure of Fiction." Beth Newman makes the argument that in *Frankenstein,* story and character become separable elements: "In other words, a story is emphatically separable form the character who first tells it; once a narrative has been uttered, it exists as a verbal structure with its own integrity, and can, like myth, think itself in the minds of men (and women). Being infinitely repeatable in new contexts, it has achieved autonomy; it now functions as a text, having been severed from its own origins, divested of its originating voice. The mark of this severance is the frame itself" ("The Frame Structure," 172).

12 Barbara Johnson, "My Monster/My Self," *Diacritics* 12, no. 2 (1982): 2.

13 Based on thorough examinations of the various manuscripts of *Frankenstein* and Mary Shelley's journal, David Ketterer asserts that "(for her account of the monster's growing awareness she studies Locke's *An Essay Concerning Human Understanding* intensively between 18 November 1816 and 8 January 1817) ... "; David Ketterer, "(De)Composing *Frankenstein*: The Import of Altered Character Names in the Last Draft," *Studies in Bibliography: Papers of the Bibliographical Society of the University of Virginia* 49 (1996), 263. Certain sections of book 2, chapters 1 and 3 of John Locke's *An Essay Concerning Human Understanding* suggest themselves as intertexts: particularly §6 in chapter 1 on the "state of a child." Brooks, in contrast, contends: "Like so much else in the story of the Monster's education through sensation, experience, and the association of ideas, his discovery of language stands within enlightenment debates about origins, coming in this instance close to the scenarios of Rousseau's *Essai sur l'origine des langues*, which sees language originating not in need but in emotion"; Peter Brooks, "What Is a Monster?" in Botting, *New Casebooks Frankenstein*, 86. For an excellent discussion of the potential reference to the polemical representation of Godwin and his political philosophy as a "monster" see again Sterrenburg, "Mary Shelley's Monster: Politics and Psyche in *Frankenstein*," 143-171. Shelley's reading of Rousseau can be documented and demonstrated through reference both to her journals and the encyclopedia article on Rousseau of her authorship; O'Rourke, "'Nothing More Unnatural': Mary Shelley's Revision of Rousseau," 543-69.

language, although the monster attains to expression and then to language in an eccentric and historically complex way. His "origin narrative" comes forth in a subsequently formed "I," experiential and subjective, and takes place not prior to but contemporaneous with the history of the European present.[14] He *originates* in Rousseau's Geneva and introduces interesting problems into it, for when the monster does appropriate the capacity for "human" speech, he almost immediately uses the capacity to narrate a history and voice a demand. The demand he voices is a rights-based claim upon a community (by way of a companion or mate). Even more interestingly, its first utterance comes in terms of a "requisition." The narration of the events of his life and his development have all been a prelude to the voicing of this demand with which he concludes his narrative:

> We may not part until you have promised to comply with my requisition. I am alone and miserable; *man* will not associate with me; but one as deformed and horrible as myself would not deny *herself* to me. My companion must be of the same species and have the same defects.[15] (411)

By demanding that another of "his species" be produced, the monster announces himself as member of a species, though he importantly lacks the requisite other members. The monster demands, in the name of community, that he be produced not only a companion but also one of the formal preconditions of his status as member of a species – that there be others. In producing the second, the Doctor will effectively create the first as species. The possibility of reproduction in the new species, attendant upon this act, however, escalates the calamity of the monster's being

14 In this, the monster both does and does not resemble the "boy of about ten," invoked by Étienne Bonnot de Condillac in his *Essay on the Origin of Human Knowledge*, who "lived among bears" in the forests between Russia and Lithuania. "It took a long time before he could utter a few words, which he still did in a very barbarous manner. As soon as he could speak, he was asked about his former state. But he could not remember any more than we can recall what happened to us in the cradle." Like that boy, the monster cannot develop his capacity for language until he finds a human example to imitate; unlike him, he is later able to narrate his previous existence; Etienne Bonnot de Condillac, *Essay on the Origin of Human Knowledge*, ed. Hans Aarsleff (Cambridge: Cambridge University Press, 2001), 88.

See Gayatri Chakravorty Spivak's definitive discussion of the role Safie plays in the humanizing of the monster's development and the daemon's attainment of literacy through the axiomatics of imperialism; Gayatri Chakravorty Spivak, *A Critique of Postcolonial Reason* (Cambridge: Harvard University Press, 1999), 138.

15 Where "man" will not associate a feminine gendered other will? Note how in this instance, the universal, abstract parlance of "one" is jarringly displaced by the feminine pronoun, announcing the immediacy, concretion, and specificity of the demand. The appearance of this gender-shift is beautifully sudden, as the masculine pronoun – so easily overheard in the parlance of a subject's rights – had not yet led to an explicit demonstration of his, the daemon's, genital viability.

such that he would not only systematically destroy all the Doctor loves but would represent a threat to mankind itself and a peril to the human community – as the Doctor puts it, a desolation of the "world" (108).

Shelley introduces a chapter break between the requisition with which the monster ends his autobiographical narrative and the declaration he voices. The monster's long narrative thus cedes in chapter 17 to a dramatic dialogue between monster and maker and then restores the narrator's position to Dr. Frankenstein. Following is the monster's declaration as reported later by him:

> The being finished speaking and fixed his looks upon me in the expectation of a reply. But I was bewildered, perplexed, and unable to arrange my ideas sufficiently to understand the full extent of his proposition. He continued, "You must create a female for me with whom I can live in the interchange of those sympathies necessary for my being. This you alone can do, and I demand it of you as a right which you must not refuse to concede." (108)

The Doctor begins this chapter by naming the monster a "being" instead of a "daemon," and one wonders if this might be an effect of the light of reason cast by what Shelley has the daemon term his "proposition." It is not reason, however, that renders the Doctor pliable but rather the quality of the story. " ... [A]nger ... had died away while he narrated his peaceful life among the cottagers . . ." (108). The pastoral scene of the monster's education and surreptitious initiation into human society allows the "being" to become an object worthy of sympathy: precisely that which he demands to be at liberty to share and the signature sentiment of the epistolary frame. The proposition that concludes the narration, however, produces uncontrollable rage. Dr. Frankenstein recounts, "and as he said this I could no longer suppress the rage that burned within me" (108). The sympathy inspired by what one might construe as the result of an identification produced by sentimental readership cannot sustain the logical consequence that the monster would draw from it, that is, his claim on the right to community – the positive freedom of a right to the exchange of sympathies with "one of his own species." This claim, the monster believes, follows as a consequence of his tale, but it inspires fear and loathing in his creator, who, despite his sympathy, refuses the analogy to the rights of the citizen and, indeed, regards that analogy as a biological threat to mankind.

Doubling Geneva *or* Is Frankenstein's Monster a Kantian?

The monster's narration of his "origins" and its culmination in his proposition, suggest Rousseau's *Origine de l'inégalité parmi les hommes* as an intertext for Shelley's novel. The monster's additional reference to traveling to the "wilds of South America" with his future mate further reinforces this connection (413).[16] Just as Rousseau's response to the Académie de Dijon resorts to the tracing of the history of "la vie de ton espèce [homme]" in order to account for the origin of inequality among men and answer the question whether it is "authorized" by natural law, the monster's gradual acquisition of language and the trajectory of his development provide a standard by which to measure the justice of his claim. Like Rousseau's early man, the monster demonstrates an innate "pity" in the first phases of his interaction with man. His initial impulse is only clouded and obscured by the brutal and uncomprehending responses with which this species of man responds to the product of the Doctor's laboratory. This line of development parallels the "progress" of reason in history charted by Rousseau in the second *Discourse*. Reason distorts the initial "sensibility" of man, which Rousseau affirms as *prior* to it. Let us recall Rousseau's terms for a moment:

> and meditating on the first and simplest operations of the human Soul, I believe I perceive in it two principles prior to reason, of which one interests us intensely in our well-being and our self-preservation, and the other inspires in us a natural repugnance at seeing any sentient Being [*être sensible*], and especially any being like ourselves [*nos semblables*], perish or suffer. It is from the association and combination which our mind is capable of making between these two Principles, without it being necessary to introduce into it that of sociability, that all the rules of natural right seem to me to flow; rules which reason is subsequently forced to reestablish on different foundations when, by its successive developments, it has succeeded [*elle est venue à bout*] in smothering nature.[17]

---

16 I concur with Jean Starobinski's insistence that Rousseau's philosophy of "natural man" is not meant to have any particular historical referent; Jean Starobinski, *Jean-Jacques Rousseau: La transparence et l'obstacle* (Paris: Gallimard, 1971), 330-55. Claude Lévi-Strauss also makes this point in *Tristes Tropiques* (New York: Atheneum, 1977), 38. Rousseau carefully sets the empirical study of man and "les livres scientifiques" to one side in his preface, beginning his answer with the inspired phrase: "Commençons donc, par écarter tous les faits ... "; Rousseau, *Oeuvres complètes*, vol. 3 (Dijon: Gallimard, 1985), 123. Rousseau's natural man is no less a concoction that Shelley's daemon (as Shelley herself notes in her encyclopedia entry). Nonetheless, one cannot therefore overlook the running presence of "facts" – proto-anthropological studies contemporary to Rousseau – in the footnotes of the first part and throughout the extended, optional endnotes.

17 Rousseau, *The First and Second Discourses*, trans. Victor Gourevitch (New York: Perennial Library, 1986), 132-33. Rousseau, *Oeuvres complètes*, vol. 3, 125-26.

This "sensibility," which predates reason and obviates the need to posit "sociability," provides the standard in Rousseau's second *Discourse* whereby the distance from a better and original nature of man can be gauged. It further proposes a model for the recuperation of this better nature through the establishment of "other foundations."[18] Reason, then, is set the task in the discourse of reestablishing, through its own methods, a prior state of affairs that the very progress of reason, as Rousseau maintains, has destroyed. The monster's narration of his history closely follows the Rousseauvian argument. He addresses his tale to the Doctor as a kind of testimony and insists that it be heard in the name of his original constitution: "By the virtues that I once possessed, I demand this from you. Hear my tale ... " (365). Pity is only extinguished in the monster, an initially sympathetic observer of human activity, by the misrecognition of the monster's resemblance to "man" – his own original pity. This introductory passage turns, meanwhile, on precisely that point in the above-cited passage from Rousseau that will exclude the daemon from "nature." He does not resemble his creator sufficiently to sustain the sympathy that he hopes to elicit. What follows is Dr. Frankenstein's response to the being's request for a hearing and, in turn, the monster's response to it.

> "Why do you call to my remembrance," I rejoined, "circumstances of which I shudder to reflect, that I have been the miserable origin and author? Cursed be the day, abhorred devil, in which you first saw light! Cursed (although I curse myself) be the hands that formed you! You have made me wretched beyond expression. You have left me no power to consider whether I am just to you or not. Begone! Relieve me from the sight of your detested form."
>
> "Thus I relieve thee, my creator," he said, and placed his hated hands before my eyes, which I flung from me with violence; "thus I take from thee a sight which you abhor. Still thou canst listen to me and grant me thy compassion." (75)

Though the monster proves himself to share in that fundamental "sensibility" of man that Rousseau describes, the limitations of the human senses bar his access to justice. Throwing his hand over the Doctor's eyes, he ironizes the possibility of a "blind" justice and literalizes the figure of a "hearing." The shift provided by Rousseau's introduction of "sensibility" as a foundation for natural law – "It appears, in effect, that if I am obliged to do no harm to my kind [*semblable*], it is less because he is a reasonable being [*être raisonnable*] than because he is a sensible being [*être sensible*]...)" –

18 Starobinski offers a dialectical reading of Rousseau's understanding of reason in the second *Discourse*; Starobinski, *La transparence et l'obstacle*, 346-47.

still excludes the monster, possessed of reason and sensibility, who cannot attain status as *un semblable* (162).

Here we encounter the problem of identity between doctor and monster. While, the Doctor and monster double one another, they also prove, in the overlapping of their positions, to be no longer identical to themselves. The work of the Doctor's hands (the creation of this ranging, destructive other) has alienated him from himself and his authorship and from the site of this alienation, he lacks the "power" – of either sensibility or reason – to judge the monster's request. The fact that his narration can move the Doctor allows the monster some footing in the Rousseauvian fiction concerning the life of the human species. However, the final step, whereby the intervention of reason would restore the lost innocence of sensibility, is roundly refused the monster by the Doctor's response to the very thought. He will not grant the monster his right to a community, either as social or species being. Neither "reason" nor "sensibility" will suffice, and Shelley's narrative underlines, as does Rousseau's second *Discourse*, the priority of the *semblable* even to the *sensible* in this struggle for recognition. Further, their failed resemblance to one another having destroyed their access to an original sensibility, the daemon and Doctor mutually destroy one another's self-identity.

The particularity of their connection to one another – never to be sufficiently defined as one of mirroring because it is precisely a *product of labor* or *act of reproduction* that is a stake – nullifies their abstract and equal value before what Rousseau might propose as reason's intervention in the history of civilization. The Doctor takes on the "cause of mankind" as the human who stands between the daemon and the final enunciation of the daemon's being. Interestingly, it is, in the last instance, the Doctor's incapacity and subsequent active refusal of the monster's proposition that causes the monster's failure to be a *semblable*.

> "I do refuse it," I replied; "and no torture shall ever extort a consent from me. You may render me the most miserable of men, but you shall never make me base in my own eyes. Shall I create another like yourself, whose joint wickedness might desolate the world? Begone! I have answered you; you may torture me, but I will never consent." (108)

The monster should by all rights inherit the rights of man and the citizen: he is possessed of sensibility and can reason on his own behalf. By virtue of both of these capacities he becomes able to voice a claim. It is precisely the voicing of his particular claim, however, that leads directly to the escalation of the Doctor's response, that is, Dr. Frankenstein's fear that the monster will also "inherit the earth" and threaten the *common* good of mankind. The monster's projected *social* being is precisely what Dr. Frankenstein has come to regard as a direct threat to his own. Further, the exponential threat posed by the monster's species-being drives the Doctor to desire to murder his creation *genocidally.* It is not the daemon alone whom the Doctor must destroy but his *race*, and this race, in turn, would already come into conceptual being through any acknowledgment of the claim that the monster voices. His claim on justice therefore persists, thereafter, and as we shall see it is this justice which haunts Dr. Frankenstein.

While it is true that the monster's narrative also details the development and history of his criminality, a contradiction emerges precisely because he cannot be recognized by the law:

> "The guilty are allowed, by human laws, bloody as they are, to speak in their own defence before they are condemned. Listen to me Frankenstein. You accuse me of murder, and yet you would, with a satisfied conscience, destroy your own creature. Oh, praise the eternal justice of man! Yet I ask you not to spare me, and then if you can, and if you will, destroy the work of your hands." (Penguin 365)

The being says that he is "content to reason" (412), and as he reasons, he finds himself to be outside of the protection of the law: though a murderer subject to "human laws," the destruction of his own being would not be comprehended as murder under those same laws. (The monster is satisfyingly sarcastic on this point.) Notably, the daemon names the laws as specifically human, and through a confusion of modification, the line could also read as follows: not necessarily the guilty, but potentially also the laws, are bloody. The daemon's drama immediately emphasizes the fact that the laws that can only identify him as a perpetrator, but not as a victim, apply to embodied subjects; beyond that they apply specifically to human bodies, the humanly embodied subject. Not the dictates of reason but the limitations of the empirically human debar the daemon's recognition before the law.

The monster's accentuation of the human embodiment upon which the laws of Geneva are contingent raises a question of justice. His demand sets the ethical tasks of reason in relief against the anthropological determination of the reasoners themselves. In this the monster turns out to be a good Kantian through circumstance; that is, by being forced, by virtue of his very embodiment, to draw a fine distinction between "pure moral philosophy" and "anthropology."[19] Indeed, the manufactured man might fare better if viewed in the light of Kantian ethics, for Kant's investigation

---

19 See Immanuel Kant, *Critique of Practical Reason*, trans. Lewis White Beck (New Jersey: Prentice Hall, 1993), 3. German: Immanuel Kant, *Werkausgabe*, vol. 7, ed. Wilhelm Weischedel (Frankfurt a.M.: Suhrkamp, 1974), 107.

of the existence of pure practical reason, obliges him to eliminate the empirical – and with it the human – from the ultimate articulation of the moral law.[20] This necessity functions as both the endpoint and prerequisite of Kantian ethics.

> This, then, is the first question: Is pure reason sufficient of itself to determine the will, or is it only as empirically conditioned that it can do so? At this point there appears a concept of causality which is justified by the *Critique of Pure Reason*, though subject to no empirical exhibition. That is the concept of freedom, and if we can now discover means to show that freedom does in fact belong to the human will (and thus to the will of all rational beings), then it will have been proved not only that pure reason can be practical but also that it alone, and not the empirically conditioned reason, is unconditionally practical.[21]

Paradoxically, the attempt to provide that the causality of freedom belongs to the human will necessitates, for Kant, that that part of the human under consideration be shorn of all empirical attributes and generalized *beyond* the human itself, that is, freedom must also belong to all rational beings. Who are they? No further elucidation is proffered and the discussion attends to the question of principles. Principles must be proven to be possessed of objective necessity and therefore must be "known a priori" (prior to any empirical testing) in order to qualify as "laws."[22] Objectivity must be distinguished from universality when determining whether a given principle can be understood as a law. That is why the pursuit of happiness cannot be a law: though universal, it is nevertheless subjectively and empirically determined. To operate as a law, a practical principle must include the human under a wider, objective rubric of necessity that can only be vouched for by reason's evidence unto itself. This also explains why the hallmark of the law is its pure formality. Kant reiterates the importance of the simultaneous narrowing and widening of the aperture in the *Foundations of the Metaphysics of Morals*:

> Since my purpose here is directed to moral philosophy (*sittliche Weltweisheit*), I narrow my proposed question to this: Is it not of the utmost necessity to construct a pure moral philosophy which is completely freed [*gesäubert*] from

---

20 "And while empirical laws may give him valuable guidance, a purely empirical theory of right, like the wooden head in Phaedrus' fable, may have a fine appearance, but will unfortunately contain no brain." Immanuel Kant, "Foundations for the Metaphysics of Morals" in *Political Writings*, ed. Hans Reiss (Cambridge: Cambridge University Press, 1991), 132.

21 Kant, *Critique of Practical Reason*, 15. German: Kant, *Werkausgabe*, vol. 7, 120.

22 Ibid., 19-20.

> everything which may be only empirical [*nur empirisch heißen mag*] and thus belong to anthropology?[23]

Responding on a fundamental level to the new disciplines in the human sciences – comparative law, in this case – developed in the earlier part of the century (for instance, by Montesquieu), Kantian ethics turn roundly away from the efforts of an empiricist universalism.[24] As Louis Althusser remarks with respect to Montesquieu's *The Spirit of the Laws*,

> The project of constituting a science of politics and history presupposes first of all that politics and history can be the object of a science, i.e., that they contain a *necessity* which the science can hope to discover.[25]

Kantian ethics takes a diametrically opposite approach, turning from politics and history to the necessity that can be demonstrated in the conceptual realm of freedom, to a formal rather than a determinate ethics. Instead of seeking out necessity sufficient to the formation of an object of knowledge within the chaos of accumulated facts, Kant frames the highest ethical imperative (understood as the pursuit of "law") in terms of establishing a necessity prior to the facts, a necessity argued to be inherent in reason. In order to avoid the contagion of the "pathologically determined" faculty of desire in this conjectured "higher faculty of desire," Kant in essence returns the question of human law to a speculative, prior stage, insisting that the critique of practical reason be analogous to mathematics.

---

23 Immanuel Kant, *Foundations of the Metaphysics of Morals and What Is Enlightenment?* trans. Lewis White Beck (New Jersey: Prentice Hall, 1997), 5. German: Kant, *Werkeausgabe*, vol. 7, 13.

24 See Louis Althusser for a discussion of the relation of global exploration, civil war in Europe, and the Reformation to the rise of the project of writing the "history of all men who have ever lived." I shall cite here one section: "these upheavals, whose echo can be heard in all the works of the period, gave the material of the scandalous tales brought back from across the seas the contagious dignity of facts real and full of meaning. What had previously been themes for compilation, extravaganzas to appease the passions of the erudite, became a kind of mirror for the contemporary unease and the fantastic echo of this world in crisis. This is the basis for the *political exoticism* (known history itself, Greece and Rome, becoming the *other world* in which the present world seeks its own image) which has dominated thought since the sixteenth century.

"Such is Montesquieu's object, too. As he says, 'The objects of this work are the Laws, the various customs, and manners of all the nations on earth. It may be said, that the subject is of prodigious extent, as it comprehends all the institutions received among mankind' [*A Defence of the Spirit of Laws* Part II: The General Idea]. It is precisely this object that distinguishes him from all the writers who, before him, had hoped to make a politics of science: For never before him had anyone had the daring to reflect on *all the customs and laws of all the nations of the world*"; Louis Althusser, *Montesquieu, Rousseau, Marx*, trans. Ben Brewster (London: Verso, 1982), 19.

25 Ibid., 20.

This analogy is based on the conviction that the empirical will "degrade" the demonstration.[26]

> Then only is reason a truly higher faculty of desire, but still only in so far as it determines the will by itself and not in the service of the inclinations. Subordinate to reason as the higher faculty of desire is the pathologically determinable faculty of desire, the latter being really and in kind different from the former, so that even the slightest admixture of impulses impairs the strength and superiority of reason, just as taking anything empirical as the condition of a mathematical demonstration would degrade and destroy [*herabsetzt und vernichtet*] its force and value."[27]

If anything, the spectacle of Mary Shelley's man-made, animate product declaring his rights amid the rigorous sublimities of Mont Blanc would seem to approach a "degraded and blasted demonstration." And yet, because the monster falls outside of the category of the strictly anthropological, his existence becomes, by default, an *instance* – a problematically intransigent *example* – of another, differently embodied, rational creature. The novel *Frankenstein*, in essence, startlingly and abruptly responds to the above-stated question: Who are these *other* rational, finite beings? Let us recall Kant:

> Everyone must admit that a law [*ein Gesetz*], if it is to hold morally (i.e. as a ground of obligation), must imply absolute necessity; he must admit that the command: thou shalt not lie, does not apply to men only as if other rational beings had no need to observe it. The same is true for all other moral laws properly so called. He must concede that the ground of obligation here must not be sought in the nature of man or in the circumstances in which he is placed [*gesetzt*] . . .[28]

The presentation of the argument moves from an assumed consensus (*jedermann muß eingestehen*) to the assertion of a critical requirement that moral laws, to be binding, must find their foundations beyond this consensus in the strictures of reason. As we shall see, these shall be laid out in terms of the formal conditioning of a "law," which I will consider as reason's relation to itself. The bindingness of law does not reside in its humanness, nor even its empirical circumstances – the world into which

26 Compare Althusser on Montesquieu to Kant on practical reason. Althusser: "We might say that their science [Hobbes, Spinoza, Grotius] is as far from Montesquieu's as the speculative physics of a Descartes is from the experimental physics of a Newton. The one directly attains in simple natures or essences the *a priori truth* of all possible physical facts, the other starts from the facts, observing their variations in order to disengage their *laws*"; Althusser, *Montesquieu, Rousseau, Marx*, 20.

27 Kant, *Critique of Practical Reason*, 24. German: Kant, *Werkausgabe*, vol. 7, 132.

28 Kant, *Political Writings*, 5. German: Kant, *Werkausgabe*, vol. 7, 13.

people are set [*gesetzt*] does not, in fact, ground the other way in which they are set up in the law [*Gesetz*].

In one sense, the humans who observe the law also witness the law's formal determination of itself and are outside of it, though simultaneously under it. The humans gather to witness this self-evidence of reason, but with the monster unleashed in Geneva, their witnessing itself is also disturbingly observed. The reader recalls Shelley's description of her first semi-conscious production ("I did not sleep, nor could I be said to think...") of the story from the "Author's Introduction":

> [the Doctor] sleeps; but he is awakened; he opens his eyes; behold, the horrid thing stands at his bedside, opening the curtains and looking on him with yellow, watery, but speculative eyes. (263-264)

If the humans gather to witness the relationship of reason to itself, the monster at large in Geneva uncannily shadows and witnesses this scene.

* * *

In Kant's ethics, the problem of an unexplored species difference is preferred to the problem of cultural or historical difference. The vagaries of inter-human differences are drawn into shadow by the umbrella concept of "the empirical." Though refusing any assertion of transcendence outside the limits of reason, Kant also refuses to anchor the principle of law in anthropological universalism. While this move to the *a priori* jurisdiction of reason would appear to skirt the political, it can also be brought into the service of a proleptic affirmation thereof. The daemon of Shelley's *Frankenstein*, in declaring his rights as another reasoning species, accepts the challenge of objective moral necessity and makes it political.[29]

If the novel *Frankenstein* inaugurates "science fiction," this is partly by its forcing of a proviso of non-empirical, *a priori* knowledge (i.e., that freedom must necessarily belong to all rational beings) onto a kind of road test. Shelley's fiction unleashes a being adequate to the category of the "reasoning non-human" – the counter-category that provides the back-

29 Note that Kant's argument forestalls the possibility that all finite rational beings might possess identical feelings – the importance of the distinction is still categorical and not circumstantial. "But suppose that finite rational beings were unanimous in the kind of objects their feelings of pleasure and pain had, and even in the means of obtaining the former and preventing the latter. Even then they could not set up the principle of self-love as a practical law, for the unanimity itself would be merely contingent [*zufällig*]"; Kant, *Critique of Practical Reason*, 25; German: Kant, *Werkausgabe*, vol. 7, 133-4. It would still not be a priori – grounded in the legislation of reason. The "empirically universal" remains "merely empirical."

ground for reason's self-evidence in Kant's ethics[30] – and follows its (narrative) progress. In this sense, the novel sets up a kind of aftermath of the *a priori* because the daemon, when he comes alive, is subject to the reign of consequences, the succession of incidents, the necessities of existence. Thus, the hulking figure moves from the background of a given, formal condition of the ethical law (*Sittengesetz*) onto the scene of the law's operation. Once participation in the *Sittengesetz* of the categorical imperative, the law of freedom, is *voiced* as a claim by the daemon, it leaves its initial formality as established in the second *Critique* by Theorem III and moves into its perhaps unintended and unexpected use. Let us recall Theorem III:

> If a rational being can think (*denken soll*) of his maxims as practical universal laws, he can do so only by considering them as principles which contain the determining grounds of the will *because of their form* and not because of their matter. (emphasis mine)

The universal objective law in Kant is powerfully formal and empty. The categorical imperative *gives* the form and that form is necessarily "identical and self-evident [*für sich klar*]." The principle of contradiction assures the jurisdiction of practical reason on formal grounds and offers anchoring in the *a priori.*

> The will is thought of as independent of empirical conditions and consequently as pure will, determined by the mere form of law, and this ground of determination is regarded as the supreme condition of all maxims.[31]

Practical reason gives the form of the universal law and "determines the will a priori only with respect to the form of its maxims" (31). It demands that any maxim of the individual will "could always hold at the same time as the principle giving universal law" (30). It establishes, in other words, the hypothetical limiting condition that the individual will must participate in the universal giving of law. (Here we have come very close to the principle of contradiction that undergirds the thinking of Rousseau's general will.) This is made clear by virtue of the necessary form that each maxim takes. How then does the daemon's demand measure up with respect to Kantian maxim-testing?

The problem with Shelley's monster is that the demand he makes – based on his participation in the inherent freedom of reasoning beings – is that he be *given* a community. The "nature" of this demand unfortunately for him entails the possibility that he become capable of reproduction. His

---

30 For a reading of the connection between monstrosity and Kant's sublime see Barbara Claire Freeman, "*Frankenstein* with Kant: A Theory of Monstrosity or the Monstrosity of Theory," in Botting, *New Casebooks Frankenstein*, 191-205.

31 Kant, *Critique of Practical Reason*, 31. German: Kant, *Werkausgabe*, vol. 7, 141.

claim, however, which I understand as a "politicization" of the critique of pure practical reason, lands the monster immediately at the crux of an unsustainable contradiction. While the monster or daemon is a reasoning being, what he demands from his participation in the community of reasoning beings is notably *doubly* empirical, because it follows along the lines of the "pursuit of happiness" (a subjective, if universal, grounding of a will's determination) and because it threatens to produce as its consequence a crisis of proliferation of material, alien *forms,* that is, a competing sphere of contingency in the precincts of the human.

The unnamed daemon demands the right to his species-being – not only "to be" a species, but paradoxically, to "become" one – which, at the moment of the declaration, is the same as producing one. In a community of reason with the human reasoners he asks to reassert his species-difference therefrom, by requisitioning his own alien community of reason. The production of these others, though utterly assimilable in the context of empirical cataloguing, complicates the purity of the formal rule of law by its relationship to embodiment and proliferation. The monster thus moves from playing a potential role in grounding a demonstrable transhuman category to exiling himself from the ethics of pure practical reason because of his kind of embodiment and its unprecedented conditions.

As mentioned parenthetically above, when viewed from one perspective, the different mechanisms for rendering the operation of the law non-arbitrary and necessary in both the case of Kant's categorical imperative and Rousseau's general will have the result of *necessarily* aligning the individual will to a more general faculty of "volition." We have considered the case in terms of the formal structure of the categorical imperative. How will it appear with reference to the general will?

Shelley's daemon, when making a demand for a community, is in the unique position – conspicuously parallel to the hypothetical regions of Rousseau's social contract – of needing to establish his participation in the *general* before attending to his being as the *particular*. The monster is (diegetically) unequivocally empirical, although his being (but not his existence) can be argued in another sense to be the supplement – the possible/potential other, finite reasoning being possessed of will – that grounds the *objective* universality of the law for Kant.[32] By insisting that he be

32 "Now this principle of morality, on account of the universality of its legislation which makes it the formal supreme determining ground of the will regardless of any subjective differences among men, is declared by reason to be a law for all rational beings in so far as they are competent to determine their actions according to principles and thus to act according to practical a priori principles, which alone have the necessity which reason de-

granted the rights attendant to human freedom, however, the daemon emphasizes and *corporeally* reiterates the disavowed physicality of the political subject of the Enlightenment and signals toward the "private sphere" of female non-subjects, slaves and servants (what might be loosely characterized as the reproductive or economically conditioned social sphere), which renders this subject possible. The formal conflation of the particular and general will is literally collapsed in the monster's body, which lacks the maintenance of a "private sphere," rendering him the perfect, supernumerary embodiment of a political fiction. The record of his criminality aside, the monster is not a viable subject largely because of his peculiar relation to the disavowed "givenness" of the existence of social groups and sexual dominance in eighteenth-century political fictions and political reason.

Interestingly enough, what is for Dr. Frankenstein the grotesque impossibility of the monster's demand points to what Althusser calls "the first encounter with a real problem" in Rousseau's *Social Contract*, that is, the existence of particular interest *groups*. In the chain of discrepancies Althusser pursues through Rousseau's articulation of the social contract, each *décalage* is occasioned by an explanatory strategy marked by the phrase "so to speak." In the last discrepancy "particular interest" is the locus of the play on words or the pivotal double entendre. "Particular interest," Althusser argues, is what Rousseau terms both the interest of the individual in isolation and that of a particular social group.[33] This double usage allows for the inclusion of a total contradiction. It causes the particular interest to be both the essence and the obstacle to the general interest because the existence of "partial societies" is said to inhibit the general interest from expressing itself.[34] The mirroring relation between the particular and general interest is thus, to follow Althusser's argument, predicated upon the exclusion of social groups. These same remain, nonetheless, an insurmountable fact of politics.[35]

---

mands in a principle. It is thus not limited to human beings but extends to all finite beings having reason and will; indeed, it includes the Infinite Being as the supreme intelligence"; Kant, *Critique of Practical Reason*, 32.

33 Althusser, *Montesquieu, Rousseau, Marx*, 151.

34 "It is therefore essential, if the general will is to be able to express itself, that there should be no partial society within the State, and that each citizen should think only his own thoughts"; Ibid., 150.

35 "This 'play' on words is once again the index of a Discrepancy: a difference in theoretical status of the isolated individual and social groups – this difference being the object of denegation inscribed in the ordinary use of the concept of *particular interest*. This denegation is inscribed in so many words in his declaration of impotence: human groups must not exist in the State. A declaration of impotence, for if they *must not* exist, that is because they *do* ex-

The monster's peculiar relationship to the possibility of acceding to a social form of being and the question of progeneration, which accompanies this possibility, also point to this *décalage* investigated in Althusser's study of Rousseau. Within the matrix of Shelley's novel, the monster is not just the sad outsider famous to the twentieth century from the cinema of James Whale. Rather, he represents a particular interest literally cut loose from any particular interest group and striving to produce one. His existence thus amounts to a total collapse of the difference between particular and general and results in a *quest for* the elided second usage of the term "particular interest." In this he impossibly embodies or figures the slip between the two uses of particular interest in Rousseau's exposition of the social contract. He is an alien but in a remarkably human way, which is to say that he is excluded from the *human in general* because of his relation to a group – a group that does not yet exist.

The monster's registration of the problem of the group thus functions as a negative index. It's true that the point is that he conspicuously lacks a group, but, as argued above, it is precisely his attempt to invoke a just cause and requisition a companion that obliterates his relation to the community of reason. He claims that his existence (as opposed to the potential of his being) is impossible alone, but the demand for a community, which he makes in declaring his rights, is conflated with a nascent total destruction of humankind. This problem shows him again in the light of a mutant growth or shadowy presence at the scene of reason's activity. Hence my motive for reading Shelley's novel against the philosophical strategy of double attributions of the human in the Enlightenment and for reading these strategies *through* it. The figure of the monster's embodiment shadows the work of reason whether that be its self-evidence (providing the form of the law) as in Kant, its intervention in the progress of inequality in history, as in Rousseau's second *Discourse*, or its provision of the field of operations that theorizes the social contract.

In the case of the social contract, one might argue that the monster is a grotesque form that emerges from what Althusser calls the "working order of the mirror categories of particular and general interest."[36] His need interrupts the purely formal designation of the particular and general wills by insisting upon the inescapability of the social group. This aspect of his need makes him a persistently relevant figure in a number of current debates, those, for instance on the status of the "enemy combatant" or protections against discrimination on the basis of sexual choice. My read-

---

ist. An absolute point of resistance which is not a fact of Reason but a simple, irreducible fact: the first encounter with a real problem after this long 'chase'"; Ibid.

36 Althusser, *Montesquieu, Rousseau, Marx*, 152.

ing of Shelley's novel could invite the reproach that it over emphasizes the role of social groups with regard to cultural and biological reproduction at the expense of the novel's sentimental content. It is true that in their tone and content, the monster's passionate outbursts more closely echo Rousseau's *Reveries of the Solitary Walker* than they do the rhetorical hairpin turns of *The Social Contract*. Consider, for example, the opening *Promenade* of the *Reveries*:

> Me voici donc seul sur la terre, n'ayant plus de frère, de prochain, d'ami, de societé que moi-même. Le plus sociable et le plus aimant des humains en a été proscrit par un accord unanime. Ils ont cherché dans les rafinemens de leur haine quel tourment pouvoit être le plus cruel à mon âme sensible, et ils ont brisé violemment tous les liens qui m'attachoient à eux. J'aurois aimé les hommes en dépit d'eux-mêmes.[37]

In myriad instances, both the daemon and his producer could be ventriloquizing the lines of Rousseau's great autobiographical text – remembering that *Frankenstein* is also comprised of a series of autobiographies.[38] And truly, the monster's declared "claim" and "requisition" are borne upon the exquisite agony that is his loneliness, his marvelously emotional, pathological, and criminal being. Nonetheless, the question remains as to why the anguished cry of the monster comes forth in such tight allusion to the Enlightenment texts championing the project of freedom; why the monster's hideous and outcast status is constantly emphasized in the novel in terms of its *singleness*; and why, ultimately, the demand to which these eventualities force the daemon results in the horrifying vision of the reproduction of an alien "species," a "race of evils" (435). In turning to the implications of the particular "chains" of incidents concatenated in Shelley's novel, my goal is not to overlook the resonances of sentimentality in the novel but to remain attentive to this resonance's inescapably *political* dimension.[39] The Doctor claims that it is in the general interest of man-

---

37 Rousseau, *Oeuvres complètes*, vol. 1, 995. I have quoted this passage in the original, because the tone and emphasis of the original more clearly evoke the urgency of Shelley's own composition than does the English of contemporary translations. "So now I am alone in the world, with no brother, neighbor or friend, nor any company left me but my own. The most sociable and loving of men has with one accord been cast out by all the rest. With all the ingenuity of hate they have sought out the cruellest torture for my sensitive soul, and have violently broken all the threads that bound me to them. I would have loved my fellow men in spite of themselves"; Jean-Jacques Rousseau, *Reveries of the Solitary Walker*, trans. Peter France (New York: Penguin Classics, 1979), 27.

38 See Barbara Johnson, "My Monster/My Self," *Diacritics* 12, no. 2 (1982): 2.

39 One need only turn to the 1996 U.S. Supreme Court's decision in the Romer v. Evans case to behold the continuing significance of the problem of the "particular" group within the juridical struggle for equal protection of the law. Following are two brief segments of the decision written by Justice Kennedy:

kind that the daemon not become the subject of a just claim, the consequences of which would jeopardize the well-being of the whole. The monster's aim is not to form a "particular interest group," however, the determining factors of his "existence" make this unavoidable for him. Thus, let us consider them at further length.

Precisely the alarming narrative of the monster "coming-into-being" speaks to the problem of *declared* existences and the issue of their purity or formal emptiness. Let us consider Althusser's contention in detail:

> The general interest: its existence has as its sole content *the declaration of its existence*. ... The same is true, in mirror form, for the particular interest. For, the general interest is no more than the mirror reflection of the particular interest. The particular interest, too, is the object of an absolute *declaration of existence*. The two declarations echo one another since they concern the same content and fulfill the same function. And they are discrepant with respect to the same reality: the interests of social groups, the object of a denegation indispensable for the maintenance in working order of the mirror categories of particular interest and general interest. Just as the general interest is a myth, whose nature is visible once it is seen in demarcation from its real double, the 'general interests' which Rousseau calls 'particular' because they belong to human groups (orders, classes, etc.) – so the 'pure' particular interest of the isolated individual (what he obtains from the constitutive origins of the state of nature) is a myth, whose nature is visible once it is seen that it has a real 'double' in the general interests of human groups that Rousseau calls

---

"Amendment 2 bars homosexuals from securing protection against the injuries that these public accommodations laws address. That in itself is a severe consequence, but there is more. Amendment 2, in addition, nullifies specific legal protections for this targeted class in all transactions in housing, sale of real estate, insurance, health and welfare services, private education, and employment.

"We must conclude that Amendment 2 classifies homosexuals not to further a proper legislative end but to make them unequal to everyone else. This Colorado cannot do. A State cannot so deem a class of persons a stranger to its laws. Amendment 2 violates the Equal Protection Clause, and the judgment of the Supreme Court of Colorado is affirmed." Romer, Governor of Colorado, et al. v. Evans et al. (94-1039), 517 U.S. 620 (1996).

Though the questions raised by my reading of the peculiar configuration of Shelley's novel remain formal, their importance to the articulation of the 14th Amendment to the U.S. Constitution, for instance, are far from irrelevant.

Commentators who read *Frankenstein* with *Paradise Lost* have alternately aligned the daemon with Adam, Satan and Eve. True to his composite nature, all of these readings are plausible and engaging. My intent here is not to force the *being* into any definite correlation. It is easy to see how he could be an Adam looking for an Eve, a Satan railing against the generative power of Dr. Frankenstein, an Eve in allusion to Book IV of *Paradise Lost* as Brooks argues (Brooks, "What Is a Monster?," 87), or a being whose relationship to the biologically and culturally reproductive ends of the family debar him from commerce with "others" and "his own kind."

> 'particular' because they dominate the State, or struggle for the conquest of its power.[40]

The monster, if read not as a mere symptom but a product, represents an existence *more verisimilar* than the mutually reflecting myths of the general and particular interests as delineated above. By *actually* embodying their collapse into one another, he exposes, in his fantastic figure, their status as myth. By synchronizing in one body the relay of their identity, he demonstrates their impossibility (he cannot live, he says, without another). His dilemma and corresponding demand stand in, to use Althusser's words, not as a "fact of Reason, but a simple irreducible fact."[41] Put differently, the monster is a fictional character whose specific conditions *body forth* the myth exposed by Althusser by offering a literal incarnation of the impossible, but formally necessary, theorization of the social contract. In this, his story does indeed become a "myth made visible" – one that plays through and exposes the fallacy of the foundations of an unmediated identity between the purely general and the purely particular. The monster's idea of escaping to the wilds of Brazil takes on an especially sardonic cast in this light, as his remove to these environs will better support the mythic framework onto which natural man had been painted as zero hour of historical man – that is, as a projection from the future.

Bride of Frankenstein

The refusal the daemon receives from the community of man drives the narrative sequence to its next necessity: a requisitioned female. In a manner comparable to the intricacy of the Doctor's and the daemon's alienating identification with one another, the possibility of the new female daemon threatens further excess and crisis. The projected female daemon introduces both the problem of sex/reproduction/genre and a contradictory redoubling of the fiction itself. It would seem that the crisis occasioned by including a "female" within the frame of a voiced political demand pushes the fiction into ever less sustainable reaches of the probable. To this attenuated probability, perhaps, we owe the endurance and hilarity of that infinite source of sequels: the bride of Frankenstein. But let us consider the impossible function of the female product or being at closer range.

After the original urge of the first creature's production, the possibility of a second one appears quite clearly as a self-conscious labor.

---

40 Althusser, *Montesquieu, Marx, Rousseau*, 152.

41 Ibid., 151.

> During my first experiment, a kind of enthusiastic frenzy had blinded me to the horror of my employment; my mind was intently fixed on the consummation [1818 edition: "sequel," 127] of my labour, and my eyes were shut to the horror of my proceedings. But now I went to it in cold blood, and my heart often sickened at the work of my hands. (434)

Whereas the first monster came into being almost as the result of an unconscious impetus (the deep, single chord struck by Professor Waldman's enunciations), the second is a tedious and minutely real bit of handiwork. The necessity under which Dr. Frankenstein stands, now responsible to the first daemon, eradicates the last vestiges of his independence. He begins to refer to himself as a slave (117) and to see himself within the frame of the monster's own exile.[42] He describes himself as "under a ban – as if I had not right to claim their sympathies – as if never more might I enjoy companionship with them [his family]" (417). The daemon's lack of rights and community has been effectively transferred to his human creator and guarantor. The dread that fills him at the thought of leaving his promise unfulfilled drives him to action, while the destructive potential of its consequences steadily escalates in his thoughts.

The after effect of the Doctor's promise to the daemon is that it both enslaves and feminizes him. As mentioned above, the second production is less delirium than conscious handiwork, and in its undertaking the Doctor now feels himself to be under scrutiny. The Doctor's focalization of himself falls increasingly under the compass of the daemon's gaze.[43] The progress of his travels has been shadowed and his double takes on a panoptical ubiquity until, finally, the threat of his creature's presence is consummated by his actual appearance:

> I trembled and my heart failed within me, when, on looking up, I saw by the light of the moon the daemon at the casement. A ghastly grin wrinkled his lips as he gazed on me, where I sat fulfilling the task which he had allotted to me. (129)

Unsuspecting, the Doctor has become the object of a scrutinizing gaze. But is he working on a bit of lace? He is seated at the task allotted to him, he is viewed from the window, working within. The male monster has isolated and domesticated the scientist who dreamt him up and built him

42 "Or (so my fond fancy imagined) some accident might meanwhile occur to destroy him and put an end to my slavery forever" (421), and "For myself there was one reward I promised myself from my detested toils – one consolation for my unparalleled sufferings; it was the prospect of that day when, enfranchised from my miserable slavery, I might claim Elizabeth and forget the past in my union with her" (422).

43 "If I were alone, would he not at times force his abhorred presence on me to remind me of my task or to contemplate its progress?" (421).

out of parts. The lines of identity and sexuation begin to tangle radically for the shock of the discovery of this witness – and witness is no longer strong enough, but rather supervisor or overseer – directly follows the pivotal passage in which the Doctor reflects on the consequences of creating the monster's female other.

The narrative of experimentation in the novel crescendos when the Doctor, breaking from his labors, falls into a waking reverie concerning the consequences of his work. In a passage that begins with the by-now inevitable conceit of *enchaînement*, Dr. Frankenstein recounts:

> As I sat, a train of reflection occurred to me which led me to consider the effects of what I was now doing. Three years before, I was engaged in the same manner and had created a fiend whose unparalleled barbarity had desolated my heart and filled it forever with the bitterest remorse. I was now about to form another being of whose dispositions I was alike ignorant; she might become ten thousand times more malignant than her mate and delight, for its own sake, in murder and wretchedness. He had sworn to quit the neighborhood of man and hide himself in deserts, but she had not; and she, who in all probability was to become a thinking and reasoning animal, might refuse to comply with a compact made before her creation. (128)

In this passage, the solitude of the Doctor's remorse burgeons into a universal threat as the stakes are raised by the attempt to imagine the female other meant to come. The late consideration of her potential for reason would be amusing enough if it weren't followed by the possibility that she would refuse participation in a compact she did not authorize – indeed, which *preceded* her creation.[44] The threat of her discretion begins to overdetermine the *train* of Frankenstein's reflections as he vacillates between the possibility that the female monster will revile the male, flee his company, despise his kind, and disappoint his hopes. The alternate fear: that the two will join ranks and reproduce. The female monster will either reproduce the crisis one more time or reproduce it exponentially. This thought drives the scene to its crisis:

> Even if they were to leave Europe and inhabit the deserts of the new world, yet one of the first results of those sympathies for which the daemon thirsted would be children, and a race of evils [1818 edition: devils] would be propagated upon the earth who might make the very existence of the species of man a condition precarious and full of terror. Had I right, for my own benefit, to inflict this curse upon everlasting generations? I had before been moved by the sophisms of the being I had created; I had been struck senseless by fiendish threats; but now, for the first time, the wickedness of my promise burst upon me; I shuddered to think that future ages might curse

---

44 As Carole Pateman has asked: "What is the (conjectural) history of the origin of the private sphere?"; Carole Pateman, *The Sexual Contract*, 6.

> me as their pest, whose selfishness had not hesitated to buy its own peace at the price, perhaps, of the existence of the whole human race.
>
> . . . I trembled and my heart failed within me, when, on looking up, I saw by the light of the moon the daemon at the casement. A ghastly grin wrinkled his lips as he gazed on me, where I sat fulfilling the task which he had allotted to me. (436)

Dr. Frankenstein now recoils at woman's work with fatal consequences. He will no longer be the creator of life but a mere instrument of its reproduction. Yet, in this role, he will endow his daemon with the prospect of patriarchal potency, which, in his bewildered fancy, then culminates directly in inter-species war. In one split-second, the Doctor's self-understanding shifts from handmaiden to evil genius deplored by future generations. Frankenstein, now "trembling with passion, tore to pieces the thing" on which he was working (436). His labor has been alienated and he lays waste to his reproductive power. The complex lines of gender and sexuation alluded to above now involve the curious circumstance that in creating the female other, the Doctor is enslaved, feminized, and rendered both an object of scrutiny and a racial/species threat to his *own*. If the first monster reveals elisions within Enlightenment political fictions, the second throws the possibility of succession right off its tracks. If the problematic of reproduction signals the impossibility of a feminine subject in Shelley's novel, the disembodied human being which must be eradicated before existing, indicates the double-bind of rights-claims when put forward by members of structurally excluded groups.[45]

The prospect of the coming-to-life of the sexed citizen brings with it a human crisis presented in the text in terms of a future race war. In this sense, Mary Shelley's narrative experiment also escapes the airless fiction of gender difference as distinct and separable from the existence of particular groups. What the monster never allows the Doctor or reader to forget is his need for others. If the staging of the scene of the monster's appeal to his producer alludes to the speculative fictions of contractarian political philosophy, then what becomes the inevitable supplement of the fiction – an intrusion in the form of the daemon's needs – pushes the novel's plot to escalation and rupture. The point at which the monster's story takes on a life of its own and reverses the Doctor's own status could also be regarded as the juncture at which (from the point of view of the

45 Here my reading draws inspiration from Spivak's remarkably succinct statement: "The very relationship between sexual reproduction and social subject-production – the dynamic nineteenth-century topos of feminism-in-imperialism – remains problematic within the limits of Shelley's text and, paradoxically, constitutes its strength"; Spivak, *Critique of Postcolonial Reason*, 138.

citizen from Geneva) the fiction of the citizen must be curbed. The manufactured being's desire must be thwarted and its potential manifestation has to revert to a *mere* fiction (the uncreated daemon whose potential remains a narration and does not "literally" burst onto the scene).

Homme or *Citoyen*?

Dr. Frankenstein's daemon looms as a body in the mirror that abstracts the rights of the citizen and elides the existence of social groups. He calls himself an Adam and asks for the afterthought of an Eve, except he asks it of his creator, who any other might call "his/our fellow man." The monster calls upon man to grant him community of "his kind." His plea scrambles the codes, however, because it requires not a formal consensus but a creative act. The act of declaration must result in a further creative act that would then establish his *species* after the fact. The notable twist on the model of the declaration of rights introduced by the daemon's demand is that it is not based on a declaration of independence, but rather on one of dependence: dependence on the private sphere or on the sustenance provided by the particular group. Here again we hear strains of the transports of Rousseau's *Revêries.*

> A fiendish rage animated him as he said this; his face was wrinkled into contortions too horrible for human eyes to behold; but presently he calmed himself and proceeded, "I intended to reason. This passion is detrimental to me, for you do not reflect that *you* are the cause of its excess. If any being felt emotions of benevolence towards me, I should return them a hundred and hundredfold; for that one creature's sake I would make peace with the whole kind! But I now indulge in dreams of bliss that cannot be realized. What I ask of you is reasonable and moderate; I demand a creature of another sex, but as hideous as myself; the gratification is small, but it is all that I can receive, and it shall content me. It is true, we shall be monsters, cut off from all the world; but on that account we shall be more attached to one another. Our lives will not be happy, but they will be harmless and free from the misery I now feel. Oh! my creator, make me happy; let me feel gratitude towards you for one benefit! Let me see that I excite the sympathy of some existing thing; do not deny my request!" (109)

The monster blames the excess of his passion on the Doctor, and in fact, the daemon's genesis is something like an animated map of the Doctor's own history of psychic excess or better, the by-product of the mechanism of his psychic economy. Paradoxically, the monster will achieve his independence from this economy by securing his avowed dependence on a being *of another sex* – the initiation of another economy. He could achieve community with humankind through a single sympathetic response, but in default of that he seeks to assure the community of his own "kind." The monster does, arguably, hold a common stake in reason with mankind, and the Doctor's immediate response to the above outburst registers this: "I felt there was some justice to his argument" (109). He shudders, however, to think of the "possible consequences of … consent" (109). The Doctor's consent could lead to the reproduction of the being and the production of an alien species. The unnamed daemon makes a compelling promise, in the passage above, for reconciliation with the general – mankind – through commerce with the particular, one creature. This, however, would necessarily take place between him and *another* – a point that the facts of the monster's embodiment can never allow to be forgotten.

It is precisely the social non-viability of the solitary monster, though figured as a *male* being, that renders him an indicator of the sexed subject. This non-viability, not surprisingly, is double. First of all, the specificity of his body, his need for and implication in a community, cannot appear under the rubric of his "reasoning being." Further, the monster's possible entrance into the jurisdiction of reason is fatally blocked by this realm's inability to account for reproduction on any level but in terms of the formal parthenogenesis of the law itself – the spawn of reason's self-consciousness and the unspoken presuppositions of the subject of politics. The existence and perpetuation of the social group (i.e., the elided "facts" of both Kant's imperative and Rousseau's contract) haunt Geneva in the form of the monster's irrepressible demand, and the daemon gives the lie to the philosophically necessary in the form of his *need.* His requisition sends up the stronghold of pure moral philosophy. He contaminates the formal exemplarity of the category of "reasoning beings" with an example that might proliferate *materially* – an innovation of form that would also reproduce – and the form of its reproduction would become its content. The problem of the monster's relationship to the law is neither properly theoretical (realm of nature in Kant) nor ethical (realm of freedom). His case both reproduces and confuses the distinction. His is an alien instantiation of that divide. The daemon's persistence as species would radically interrupt the *givenness* of nature because he is not given in nature though he gives himself before an idea of the law through his own actions. As an instance before the law, the monster's embodiment parodies both the pure theoretical and pure ethical realms of reason.

Victor Frankenstein can hear the justice of his claim (as an ideal citizen), but cannot grant him the corollary rights of man: the protection of the necessities of his life. In the "series of his being," as an unfinished citizen, the daemon comes to figure something akin to the "unreal universality" of the rights-bearer in Karl Marx's analysis of the *Declaration of the Rights of Man and the Citizen.*

> Der vollendete politische Staat ist seinem Wesen nach das *Gattungsleben* des Menschen im *Gegensatz* zu seinem materiellen Leben. Alle Voraussetzungen dieses egoistischen Lebens bleiben *außerhalb* der Staatssphäre in der *bürgerlichen Gesellschaft* bestehen, aber als Eigenschaften der bürgerlichen Gesellschaft. Wo der politische Staat seine wahre Ausbildung erreicht hat, führt der Mensch nicht nur in Gedanken, im Bewußtsein, sondern in Wirklichkeit, im Leben ein doppeltes, ein himmlisches und ein irdisches Leben, das Leben im *politischen Gemeinwesen*, worin er sich als *Gemeinwesen* gilt, und das Leben in der *bürgerlichen Gesellschaft*, worin er als *Privatmensch* tätig ist, die anderen Menschen als Mittel betrachtet, sich selbst zum Mittel herabwürdigt and zum Spielball fremder Mächte wird. Der politische Staat verhält sich ebenso spiritualistisch zur bürgerlichen Gesellschaft wie der Himmel zur Erde ...[46]

> The perfected political state is, by its nature, the *species-life* (*Gattungsleben*) of man as opposed to his material life. ... Where the political state has attained to its full development, man leads, not only in thought, in consciousness, but in *reality*, in *life*, a double existence – celestial and terrestrial. He lives in the *political community* (*politisches Gemeinwesen*), where he regards himself as a *communal being* (*Gemeinwesen*), and in *civil society* (*bürgerliche Gesellschaft*) where he acts simply as a *private individual* (*Privatmensch*), treats other men as means, degrades himself to the role of a mere means, and becomes the plaything of alien powers. The political state, in relation to civil society, is just as spiritual as is heaven in relation to earth ...[47]

Very much in tune with Marx's analysis, Shelley's *Frankenstein* renders a specifically modern dilemma of embodiment and the monster walks the earth as a disassociated *species being* inopportunely individual and adrift. In his figure he comprehends man and citizen at once, but can no more unify these identities than does the *Declaration.*

The daemon's attempt to succeed to the rights of man brings to mind the historical reiterations and amendments of these declared rights by political movements which have fought the historical exclusions of the "universal."[48] The narrative course run by the *daemon* breaks off, and it is

---

46 Karl Marx, "Zur Judenfrage," in *Studienausgabe Band I Philosophie*, ed. Fetscher (Frankfurt a.M.: Fischer Taschenbuch Verlag, 1990), 41.

47 Karl Marx, "On the Jewish Question," in *The Marx-Engels Reader*, second edition. ed. Robert C. Tucker (New York: W.W. Norton, 1978), 33-34.

48 "This part (which inevitably becomes a *party*: the party of the universal, or of the abolition of particularities and classes) presents itself, then, not just as the most active mouthpiece of the citizenry, but as that fraction which is capable of presenting its own emancipation as the *criterion* of general emancipation (or as that fraction which, in continuing in slavery and alienation, inevitably entails the unfreedom of all). This, as we know, is what has been presented successively or simultaneously in the political discourse and practice of proletarians, women, colonized and enslaved peoples of colour, sexual minorities ... And these examples go to show that, in reality, the whole history of emancipation is not so much the history of the demanding of unknown rights as of the real struggle to enjoy rights which *have already*

in virtue of its breaking off that his place within the narrative signals to classes and collectivities posed at the limit of politics. The daemon's narrative existence pulls its reader, like the monster his maker, toward the irreducible fact of reason in difference and the hope for a composite equality, just as his dilemma drags the paradoxes of reason into political meaning.

---

been declared," Étienne Balibar, "Three Concepts of Politics: Emancipation, Transformation, Civility," in *Politics and the Other Scene* (New York: Verso, 2002), 6.

Chapter Two

Generating Universals

> ... so wie auch sonst, wenn man ihm (der Gang menschlicher Dinge) im großen betrachtet, darin fast alles paradox ist.
>
> ... as is often the case, if we regard it (the course of things human) in general, almost everything is paradoxical. - Immanuel Kant
> Matter imposes form upon form.
> – Richard Serra

The monster's dilemma illumined what is often referred to as the "formality of Kantian ethics"; for, though Kant's ethics make a powerful claim on objective universality, questions do arise: How and when could one be sure that one's maxim was "universalizable?" Is the principle of contradiction alone adequate to an ethics? How does one make the cross from reasoned reflection to embodied being? Interestingly, the monster's claim to participation in the universal also entailed a demand *for matter*. The only social recognition he could imagine required an act of making, a provision, but this very need introduced the possibility of reproduction run amok, of the emergence of a new and competing species or form that would challenge the universality of the law. The monster could run the test of Kant's ethics but he fails as a subject, because he can't sustain himself bereft of any community. In his instance, the relation between form and matter and questions of reproducibility emerged in a new way as a problem fundamental to enlightenment ethics and politics.

With *Critique of Judgment*, Kant had himself proposed to bridge the gap opened by the different forms of necessity presented by moral law and natural law in his account. The third *Critique* thus moves away from the broader inclusivity of practical reason maintained in the arguments of the 2nd – those same broader categories of reasoning being which temporarily housed the monster's legitimacy – and narrows the focus to planetary man *in situ*, the subject of aesthetic judgment in a very particular sense. The third *Critique* thus presents itself with the challenge of suturing man as moral agent into his concrete existence amidst natural laws. In this effort too, a sheer formality remains one of the hallmarks of Kant's argument, though in this case, it is the materiality of the natural organism that will come to be defined solely in terms of its *form* as an organized being. As Kant asserts in the second introduction to the work, with *Critique of Judgment* he will address the possibility that the incommensurable forms of universality represented by natural and moral law might be bridged through the critique of judgment's own special principle – the purposiveness of nature for judgment – though as his reader discovers, this can only take place in the non-determinative mode of reflective judgment.[1]

Reflective judgment is defined as the judgment that starts from a given particular but must seek the general or universal category under which it would fall. Reflective judgment thus *seeks the universal* from the particular, finds the species where only an individual being exists.[2] Within the curious logic of its inductive movement, reflective judgment takes on an unusual relationship to issues of generation and matter. Conversely, the form of the natural organism itself will come to encode judgment's own reflexivity with it very mode of embodiment. Once again, we run across paradoxes attendant to Enlightenment attempts to correlate the mode of its reasoned argument – self-evidence – with the life of embodied beings. *Critique of Judgment* provides an enormously instructive station for consideration in this regard, since with reflective judgment the systematization of nature and the systematic presentation of critique itself – its own principle of composition – cross over into each other's terrain, or more aptly, co-generate that terrain and, through self-reference and reflection, produce a universal and necessary model of cultural history.[3]

---

1 Immanuel Kant, *Critique of Judgment*, trans. Werner S. Pluhar (Indianapolis: Hackett Publishing Co., 1987), 14-15. German: Immanuel Kant, *Kritik der Urteilskraft*, ed. Wilhelm Weischedel (Frankfurt am Main: Suhrkamp-Taschenbuch Wissenschaft, 1974), 83-84. For longer passages I have often provided only Pluhar's English with some references to Kant's German in brackets. I will cite the German in its entirety where I wish to draw particular attention to the wording of the passage.

2 "Ist aber nur das Besondere gegeben, wozu sie das Allgemeine *finden soll*, so ist die Urteilskraft bloß *reflektierend*." (87) An awkward translation that retains the operative word "sollen" would run: "If, however, only the particular is given, to which the general *should be found*, then the judgment is merely *reflective*." Unlike determinative judgment, which progresses from universal to particular, subsuming particulars under a given generality, reflective judgment is called into service where a particular is given for which no universal is in evidence.

3 The place of history in Kant's philosophy can arguably only be asserted through a motivated exegesis of his works. For an extended discussion of the problem see Yirmiahu Yovel, *Kant and the Philosophy of History* (Princeton: Princeton University Press, 1980). For

A Special Principle is Necessary for Critique

Kant reiterates the importance of drawing proper distinctions at many junctures. In the *Prolegomena*, he commences his effort to render the discoveries of the *Critique of Pure Reason* more germane to popular understanding by insisting that the project of presenting (*darstellen*) knowledge as science (*Erkenntnis als Wissenschaft*) lies in the drawing and maintaining of exact distinctions. What is decisive is to find "*das Unterscheidende*," that which distinguishes or differentiates and which is absolutely peculiar to a given form of cognition: "was sie mit keiner andern gemein hat, und was ihr also *eigentümlich* ist, genau zu bestimmen." (What a cognition shares with no other and is thus *peculiar* to it. [Translation modified.])[4] Here the claim is that there must be some point of distinction to justify an inquiry into knowledge and that this inquiry must constitute a unique territory, utterly distinguishable from any other, else all the boundaries between science would run together and become confused. In the case of the *Prolegomena*, the primary threat of such a loss of defintion is presented by pure mathematics, because they too proceed from *a priori* knowledge. The work of philosophy cannot begin before it distinguishes itself from mathematics. Once Kant reminds his reader of the difference between the two that he had established in *Critique of Pure Reason*, he can proceed. Similarly, as we shall see in the case of the later *Critique of Judgment*, judgment, which itself specializes in mediating between the particular (*besonder*) and general (*allgemein*), must also be possessed of a special principle if there is to be any meaningful embarkation on such a critique.

In the first, unpublished introduction to *Critique of Judgment*, Kant repeats this desiderata. In his note to the first section, entitled "On Philoso-

---

Yovel one crucial aspect of the problem is the possibility of a "history of reason." Yovel contextualizes the issue as follows in his introduction: "The philosophers of the Age of Reason, starting with Descartes and following Plato, saw reason as eternal, non-temporal, and not bound by cultural and sociological factors. Even the limits of reason (when admitted) were to be understood *sub specie aeternitatis*. This led to a view of history as a contingent, empirical affair, without relational import in itself. Whatever is *Geschichte* is thereby mere *Historie*.... The nascent historicism of the eighteenth century challenged this classic view. The problem was not just to admit the rational import of history, but to supply it with a systematic ground" (3). For a discussion of the shift toward a philosophy of historical process in relation to secularization and the absolutist state see Reinhart Koselleck, "Modernity and the Planes of History," in *Futures Past: On the Semantics of Historical Time* (Cambridge, Mass.: MIT Press, 1985), 3-20.

4 Immanuel Kant, *Prolegomena To Any Future Metaphysics That Will Be Able To Come Forward as a Science*, trans. Paul Carus, extensively revised by James W. Ellington in *Philosophy of Material Nature* (Indianapolis: Hackett Publishing Company, 1985), 11. German: Immanuel Kant, *Werkausgabe in 12 Bänden*, vol. 5 (Frankfurt am Main: Suhkamp Taschenbuch, 1968), 124.

phy as A System" he remarks: "Much depends on defining philosophy precisely, as to its parts." (387, Translation modified, 11) In the case of *Critique of Judgment*, a precise rendering of the relation of parts to whole designates an unusually polyvalent question, since the critique will largely be dedicated to the question of the relation of part to whole in the human observation of natural organisms. The specific form of the living organism, which will come to be defined as a *Naturzweck* (an appellation that already hints at a curious splicing together of two distinct domains in Kant's philosophy), will be presented as possible for human cognition only through the assumption of the whole as preceding the parts, that is, the presupposition of systematic totality.[5] Just as Kant will conclude the first introduction by addressing the need for systematic totality within critical philosophy, the reader comes to be aware of an unusual resonance and mobility in the basic terms Kant uses to introduce the critique. Not only must philosophy be predicated on systematicity but experience is only possible through the presupposition of systematicity which in turn is precisely the special principle of judgment.

A number of spheres of systematicity emerge over the course of the first introduction: philosophy's system, the system of the higher cognitive powers, and finally the system presented to our observation by the organization of natural organisms. This latter form of systematicity is predicated on the primordial principle of judgment which Kant initially phrases in two distinct ways: "nature as *art*" and "the *technic of nature*" ("The original (*ursprünglich*) and peculiar (*eigentümlich*) concept that arises (*entspringende*) from judgment is that of nature as *art*; in other words, it is the concept of the *technic of nature* regarding its *particular* [*besonder*] laws." (393, 17). One can already appreciate the generative aspect of judgment in this pivotal enunciation: the repetition of the root *springen* here emphasizes judgment's principle as one of a powerful origination: the spontaneous emergence – springing forth – of the conception of nature as techinically formed.

At the same time, though judgment is found to have a special principle of its own, one of its further peculiarities is that it is not an independ-

5 A note on the translation of *Naturzweck*. As Pluhar points out: "Since organisms are judged as purposes but also as products of nature, Kant calls them *natural purposes*, as distinguished from 'purposes of nature,' which implies an (intentional) final purpose for nature as a whole (Ak. 378)." *Kant, Critique of Judgment*, lxxviii. *Ein Zweck* (an aim, end, object, purpose, design) calls to mind the willing agency examined in Kant's practical philosophy, while *Natur* [nature] cleary refers to the objects of experience which comprise the purview of Kant's theoretical philosophy. With this word compound Kant already signals his ambition to investigate phenomena that appear to mediate between the two distinct parts of his philosophy. At the same time, *Naturzweck* refers to what in other, more general discussions in the history of science would be called an "organism."

ent faculty as are reason and understanding: "Yet judgment is a very special [*besonderes*] cognitive power, not at all independent... [F]or judgment is merely an ability to subsume under concepts given from elsewhere." (392, 15) Judgment *only connects*, though as we will discover in *Critique of Judgment*, judgment's ostensible limitation – that of merely giving reference – also proves remarkably expansive. It's basic dependence upon the ideas and concepts given by reason and understanding does mean, though, that in the designation of its special principle, judgment itself must subdivide. It is judgment in its reflective capacity, *reflective judgment*, that requires its own critique, not the judgment that merely operates to subsume particulars under given concepts. In this, the mobility of terminology mentioned above comes to the fore once again, since Kant points out that when judgment merely subsumes, it acts *mechanically*, but where it reflects on the very possibility of conceptual designation – that which constitutes the specific activity of reflective judgment – judgment, like the systematic nature it presupposes, acts *technically*. Were it merely to subsume given particulars under given concepts, judgment would have to be seen as an instrument or tool, but in its reflective mode judgment must become in some sense autonomous and find a universal not in evidence. (402, 26) As will become clear, this delimits reflective judgment's sphere of operation to the subjective, but also extends the range of its capacity to a considerable degree, since judgment's presupposition concerning the systematicity of nature also establishes a mirroring relation between nature's technicity and judgment's own.

While judgment only connects, or refers, it performs the important function of providing the liason between a particular instance and a general rule. In this it does not gain any new territory for doctrine but serves specifically as the activity of system-making or engendering itself. The system will arise through connections and in turn will ground the possibility of drawing a connection. Hence, once judgment assumes that nature must be so organized as to conform to our judgment's penchant for systematizing and rubricating, as Kant puts it "zum Behuf der Urteilskraft" [*zum Behuf*: "for the sake of" but also, "for the end, purpose or use of judgment"] it can proceed, even in the absence of a concept, because we must presuppose our capacity to ascend from the particular to the general for experience to be possible at all. Notably, at this point of Kant's argument in the first introduction, reflective judgment also takes on a pervasive power within the circularity of the argument. Judgment's principle of systematicity within nature cannot be ascribed to experience, because the presupposition of nature's systematicity is itself the condition of possibility for experience.

> Auf Rechnung der Erfahrung kann man ein solches Prinzip auch keinesweges schreiben, weil nur unter Voraussetzung desselben es möglich ist, Erfahrungen auf systematische Art anzustellen. (23)

> Experience, too, can in no way be credited with [offering us] such a principle, because only by presupposing this principle can we engage in experiences in a systematic way. (399)

Providing the primordial origin of the possibility of a system as opposed to a mere aggregate (the outcome posed by the chance that particulars could not ever be subsumed under general concepts, principles, and rules), judgment, offering its structuring presupposition of nature as *art* or a technic of nature, constitutes a making which one could characterize as purely formal. It provides a matrix, except that it is no place – connectivity or referential relation as such – and it generates systems by assuring their form even when the eventual determination of the form remains unknown. To this extent, though it is not independently productive, its reflection forwards the investigation of nature.

> Also macht sich die Urteilskraft selbst a priori die *Technik der Natur* zum Prinzip ihrer Reflexion, ohne doch diese erklären noch näher bestimmen zu können… (26)

> Hence judgment itself makes a priori the *technic of nature* [a] principle for its reflection. But it can neither explain this technic nor determine it more closely… (402)

Judgment itself *makes* a principle for its reflection and it makes such a principle for itself. Throughout *Critique of Judgment* reflexive usage underscores the self-referentiality of reflective judgment's activity but also points to the difficult-to-describe, almost virtual productivity of its reflection. It actively produces both its own possibility and also that of experience. The arrival at judgment's own peculiar principle in the last of the three *Critiques* thus in no way countermands its basic anteriority.

Correlating General and Particular

One remarkable trait possessed by relective judgment in Kant's account remains the bidirectionality of its movement between particular and general or universal (*allgemein*). As noted above, this facility derives from the conditioning grounds of the assumption that nature forms a system. As the activity of subsumption as such, judgment clearly relates to problems of taxonomy and notably the first introduction to *Critique of Judgment* dedicates sustained attention to the designation and organization of the higher faculties themselves as well as to the project of producing orders of classification for nature. Indeed, questions of taxonomy lead Kant to engage in a moment of reflection on language usage in which he speculates on how best to use the term "specify" with respect to the logical activity of systematizing empirical laws.

> … we must, if we proceed empirically and ascend from the particular to the universal, *classify* the diverse, i.e., compare several classes, each falling under a definite concept; and, when these classes are complete[ly enumerated] in terms of their common characteristic, we must subsume them under higher classes (genera), until we reach the concept containing the principle of the entire classification (and constituting the highest genus). On the other hand, if we start from the universal concept, so as to descend to the particular by a complete division, we perform what is called the *specification* of the diverse under a given concept, since we proceed from the highest genus to low genera (subgenera or species) and from species to subspecies. Instead of saying (as we do in ordinary speech) that we must make specific the particular that falls under a universal, it would be more correct to say, rather, that we *make the universal concept specific* [*spezifiere den allgemeinen Begriff*] by indicating the diverse [that falls] under it. For the genus is (logically considered) as it were the matter, or the crude [*roh*] substrate, that nature processes into particular species and subspecies by determining it multiply; and so we can say that nature makes itself specific in terms of a certain princple (or in terms of the idea of a system), by analogy with how teachers of law use this term when they talk about the specification of certain raw [*roh*] material [*Materien*]. (402-403, 27-28)

Die Nature spezifiziere sich selbst nach einem gewissen Prinzip. "Nature specifies itself according to a certain principle" [Translation modified.] In this passage, what could be construed as the more formal and universal (genera as opposed to species) suddenly becomes the material which *takes on* form through subdivision – the most formal has now paradoxically emerged as raw substrate. Generation becomes specification and with this stroke classification may no longer be strictly distinguishable from a productive generation of forms; nor the thought of naming necessarily divorced from the thought of making. In a sense which will only become fully clear when we turn to a discussion of aesthetic judgments, in its presuppostion of nature as *art* and as forming a system, reflective judgment makes a kind of claim on nature, by asserting that it "cannot undertake to *classify* all of nature in terms of its empirical variety unless it presupposes that nature itself *makes* its transcendental laws *specific* in terms of some principle" but, at the same time, judgment only makes this claim for itself. It cannot aver that nature is organized according to law for its own (judgment's) sake but it also cannot proceed without assuming this. (403, 28)

With these opening arguments from the first introduction, Kant arrives at the central figure that will transit between the two distinct halves of *Critique of Judgment*, *Zweckmäßigkeit*.

> For we call something purposive if its existence seems to presuppose a presentation [*Vorstellung*] of that same thing; [and] natural laws that are constituted, and related to one another, as if judgment had designed them for its own need[s] are [indeed] similar to [the cases where] the possiblity of [certain] things presupposes that these things are based on a presentation [*Vorstellung*] of them. (404)

The classificatory generativity which judgment takes as an analogy to its own activity, and by which it can forge a system of natural laws, imputes technical agency to nature while also providing judgment with a reflection of its own activity. Attending once again to the use of reflexive verbs in the third *Critique*, the following sentence can be read in two ways: "Also denkt sich die Urteilskraft durch ihr Prinzip eine Zweckmäßigkeit der Natur, in der Specifikation ihrer Formen durch empirische Gesetze." Pluhar Translation: "Hence judgment, by means of its principle, thinks of nature as purposive, in [the way] nature makes its forms specific through empirical laws." Though we could also say that "judgment thinks itself a purposiveness of nature." It may be for this reason that in its composition, *Critique of Judgment* seems charged with the need to spend a considerable amount of time describing its own configuration and principle of subdivision. It, too, appears to generate itself through subdivision. In many ways, the exposition of its structure undertaken in the two introductions constitutes its very purpose while at the same time this basic self-reflexivity also makes reference to a vast conception, not only the power to connect particular to universal, but also to reflect the generative formation of nature itself.[6]

Introducing *Critique of Judgment*

Another signal of the importance of correctly characterizing the structure and composition of *Critique of Judgment* and can be seen in Kant's revision of the long first introduction into the shorter introduction that is then published with the work in 1790.[7] The final version of the introduction proves less concerned with judgment in its relation to systematic totalities (a concern strongly reinforced in both the aesthetic and teleological sections of the critique) than with an exposition of the importance and challenge of the divide between the theoretical and the practical in philosophy. The second section of the second introduction, which has no precedent in

6 *Prolegomena*, 39. German: *Werkausgabe*, vol 5, 161.

7 For a sustained discussion of the record of Kant's composition of *Critique of Judgment*, its reference to debates contemporary to it and the relation of its genesis to the work's central concerns see John H. Zammito, *The Genesis of Kant's Critique of Judgment* (Chicago: University of Chicago Press, 1992).

the first, further expounds the structural principle that both necessitates and impells the introduction of such a critique (of judgment).[8] Here the principle of systematicity is not so much at stake as what systematicity allows us to do, and it is here that Kant draws the well-known figure of an unbridgeable abyss between the two parts of his own project of critique.

Kant bases the distinction he draws between the theoretical and the practical on two "kinds of concepts" (*zweierlei Begriffe*), the concept of nature and the concept of freedom.[9] In contrast to these fixed domains, the area covered by the critique of judgment would constitute an indeterminate ground (*irgend einen Boden*) – not a domain. The existence of such a critique is nonetheless supported by an analogy to the legislative activity of the other two cognitive powers (understanding and reason) and judgment must be possessed of its own special principle.

> Even though such a principle would lack a realm (*Feld*) of objects as its own domain (*Gebiet*), it might still have some territory (*irgend einen Boden*); and this territory might be of such a character that none but this principle might hold it. (16) [10]

Judgment errs in an indeterminate terrain in which, however, it alone is valid (*geltend sein möchte*).[11] Indeed, to the extent that it enjoys jurisdiction, it enjoys that jurisdiction over indeterminacy itself; and judgment will be-

---

8 Zammito, *The Genesis of Kant's Critique of Judgment*, 264-267.

9 As Ernst Cassirer glosses it: "According to the fundamental ideas of the critical theory, nature and freedom, the is and the ought, are permanently separated"; Ernst Cassirer, *Kant's Life and Thought*, trans. James Haden (New Haven and London: Yale University Press, 1981), 272.

10 For longer passages I have often provided only Pluhar's English with some references to Kant's German in brackets. I will cite the German in its entirety where I wish to draw particular attention to the wording of the passage.

11 "Boden" might also be translated as "soil" which would allow for meaningful connections to Kant's reference to the "original seeds" of human knowledge in the *Prolegomena*. In Heidegger's reading of Kant's "ground-laying" of metaphysics the dilemma is pushed even further back to what one might imagine as a "growing" of the ground. Heidegger: "Nothing can be presupposed on behalf of the problematic of the possibility for original, ontological truth, least of all the *factum* of the truth of the positive sciences. On the contrary, the ground-laying must pursue a priori synthesis exclusively in itself, pursue it to the seed [*Keim*] which provides its ground and which allows that synthesis to develop into what it is (allows it to be possible in essence). ... From the clear insight into the peculiarity of a laying of the ground for metaphysics, Kant says of the *Critique of Pure Reason*: 'This work is difficult and demands a reader resolved to think himself gradually into a system into which nothing yet lies at its ground as given except for reason itself, and [who] thus seeks to develop knowledge from its original seeds without seeking the support of any fact.'" Martin Heidegger, *Kant and the Problem of Metaphysics*, trans. Richard Taft (Bloomington: Indiana University Press, 1990), 12. The Kant citation in this passage refers to: *Prolegomena zu einer jeden künftigen Metaphysik*, § 4.

come indispensable precisely because of its relative groundlessness. Though in the *Prolegomena*, Kant had asserted the absolute necessity of demarcating clear territories, judgment presents the challenge of its dependency (much like Dr. Frankenstein's daemon) and lands upon the contradiction of an "indeterminate territory." For this reason, it can never provide an object for doctrinal philosophy but only an occasion for critique preparatory to such a philosophy. To this extent, *Critique of Judgment* becomes an instance of critique *par excellence* in that it presents a special task to critique alone. In keeping with its basic reflexivity, judgment presents its own doubling – a peculiarly special principle that will ever remain before the threshold of philosophy.

* * *

Though no bridge can be thrown across the gulf that divides the two domains, nature and freedom, the shifting terrain of judgment does provide the scene of a transition between the two established areas. Kant asserts that concepts of nature (theoretical philosophy) cannot legislate for the domain of freedom (practical philosophy) but that we must nonetheless assume a unidirectional line of influence from the practical to the theoretical, that is, that freedom can be achieved in nature.

> The concept of freedom determines nothing with regard to our theoretical cognition of nature, just as the concept of nature determines nothing with regard to the practical laws of freedom; and to this extent it is not possible to throw a bridge from one domain to the other. And yet, even though the bases that determine the causality governed by this concept of freedom (and by the practical rule contained in this concept) do not lie in nature, and even though the sensible cannot determine the supersensible in the subject, yet the reverse is possible (not, indeed, with regard to our cognition of nature, but still with regard to the consequences that the concept of freedom has in nature); and this possibility is contained in the very concept of a causality through freedom, *whose effect is to be brought about in the world [but] in conformity with formal laws of freedom.* (35-36, 107-108, emphasis mine)[12]

In this unidirectional line of influence, Kant marks the first passage in which the "formality" of the laws of freedom cross the divide.

Purposiveness, or *Zweckmäßigkeit*, presents the form that functions as the node of correspondence between different forms of reflection.[13] It is

12 Page numbers in brackets refer first to the English text and then to the German.

13 Cassirer offers the following philological remark on the word "purposiveness" (*Zweckmäßigkeit*): "The linguistic usage of the eighteenth century construes 'purposiveness' in a wider sense: it sees in the term the general expression for every harmonious unification of the parts of a manifold, regardless of the grounds on which this agreement may rest and

important to note that the concept of purposiveness, so essential to the transition between domains, appears in the two halves of the third *Critique* in an assymetrical way: on the one hand because it is confined (aesthetic) and on the other in exile (teleological). The particular ways in which its powers are circumscribed actually highlight the important capacities of the imagination which its use sets into motion.

The difference between teleological and aesthetic judgment lies in the *exact way* in which a concept is lacking. Aesthetic judgment lacks a concept due to its reference to the subjective (feelings of pleasure and displeasure). Teleological judgment, on the other hand (usually annexed to the domain of theoretical philosophy), is in this case forced to proceed with special principles provided by reflective judgment and only lacks a concept as an exception to its rule. Kant explains that aesthetic judgment is appropriate to the critique of judgment, whereas the teleological judgment appears in the third *Critique* as if by default.

> . . . [A]esthetic judgment is a special power [*ein besonderes Vermögen*] of judging things according to a rule, but not according to concepts. Teleological judgment is not a special [*kein besonderes Vermögen*] power, but is only reflective judgment as such [*überhaupt*] proceeding according to concepts (as it always does in theoretical cognition), but proceeding, in the case of certain natural objects, according to special principles [*der besonderen Prinzipien*], namely, according to principles of a power of judgment that merely reflects upon but does not determine objects. Hence, as regards its application, teleological judgment belongs to the theoretical part of philosophy; because of its special principles which are not determinative (as would be required in a doctrine), it must also form a special part [*einen besonderen Teil*] of the critique. (35, 105-6)

As can be seen in the repetition of the adjective *besondere* in this passage, any instance of judging that begins from the particular (*das Besondere*) tends to continue to generate particularity at the formal level through subdivision in the critique.[14]

Aesthetic judgment most aptly reveals the principle whereby reflective judgment operates and teleological judgment, in certain cases, appropriates or mimics this operation. As Kant puts it: "Independent natural

---

the sources from which it may stem. In this sense the word represents merely the transcription and German rendering of that concept which Leibniz, in his system, signified by the expression 'harmony.' A totality is called 'purposive' when in it there exists a structure such that every part not only stands adjacent to the next but its special import is dependent on the other. Only in a relationship of this kind is the totality converted from a mere aggregate into a closed system, in which each member possesses its characteristic function; but all these functions accord with one another so that altogether they have unified, concerted action and a single overall significance." (*Kant's Life and Thought*, 287).

14 As Cassirer states, "The relation of the universal and the particular is forded into the center of the inquiry by the definition of judgment itself." (*Kant's Life and Thought*, 283).

beauty reveals [*entdeckt*] to us a technic of nature that allows us to represent nature as a system in terms of laws whose principle we do not find anywhere in our understanding." Eckart Förster emphasizes the indispensable and singular role played by natural beauty for the possibility of teleological judgment: "We must note that it is not reason's own systematic tendencies, nor any teleological reflections, but *natural beauty* that discloses this principle ... " also pointing out that Kant repeatedly insists that "the principle of a formal purposiveness of nature is disclosed *solely* by aesthetic judgments concerning *natural beauty*."[15] In this sense too, we could recall that Goethe may have at least once proved himself a profound, if willful, reader of Kant, when he expressed his pleasure in finding in the *Critique of Judgment* "artistic and natural production handled the same way; the powers of aesthetic and teleological judgment mutually illuminating each other."[16]

Just as aesthetic judgment, however, determines only the judge by revealing the harmonious play of the faculties, teleological judgment in these particular instances, rules only itself. In this capacity, it does, though, allow for the heuristic use of analogy in testing hypotheses: the possibility for a virtual experiment in concepts – the generation of concepts and their potential applicability. In one sense, the transitional space of possibility opened up by Kant's third *Critique* consists of a hall of mirrors. The operation of reflective judgment both suspends the determination of the particulars it strives to conceptualize while simultaneously indicating the (infinite) character of the supersensibles which give form to the law of its operation. From this we see that the introductory comments in which Kant describes the divisions he has made in writing the *Critique of Judgment* are crucial to understanding the peculiar and often radically metamorphic character of its object.

Already the question as to whether judgment should be qualified as theoretical or practical opens points of contact between the supersensible "freedom" and sensible intuitions in nature. As Jacques Derrida has argued, it is indeed the suspension caused by this gap that prepares the possibility for the project of critique itself:

> It is in the critique that, precisely, the critical suspension is produced, the *krinein*, the in-between, the question of knowing whether the theory of

15 Förster Eckart, *Kant's Final Synthesis* (Cambridge: Harvard University Press, 2000), 8.

16 Cited in Cassirer, *Kant's Life and Thought*, trans. James Haden (New Haven and London: Yale University Press, 1981), 273.

judgment is theoretical or practical, and whether it is then referred to a regulatory or constitutive instance.[17]

Derrida's reading emphasizes the simultaneity with which the production of the suspension *is* critique, the need to conceive of the two at once, though it would be more convenient to consider them discreetly or consolidate them in a practicable vocabulary that relies on the spatial metaphor in Kant. Indeed, by relying on the figure of an architectonics, one can avoid the difficult question of time within the critical philosophy's exposition. As we shall see, both the aesthetic and teleological sections of *Critique of Judgment* conjure with events in time, and the *Naturzweck* will unify synchronic and diachronic registers through the figure it provides of a structural whole. Unlike Mary Shelley's "Author's Introduction" in which she describes the basis of her authorship as the emergence of a succession of images, however, Kant's critique will consistently present itself as a structure not significantly determined by temporal succession, but rather as necessitated by various questions of subdivision. Nonetheless, *Critique of Judgment* will both define and reflect upon precisely those problems of becoming-in-time which present themselves to our thought: acts of the will and the observation of growth and reproduction in natural forms.

Aesthetic Judgment and the Generative Aspect of its Autonomy

One of the most troublesome tasks for the exposition of aesthetic judgment in *Critique of Judgment* is the question of its empirical status, for aesthetic judgment is said to proceed from a singular experience or experiment while simultaneously generating a rule. It therefore operates in the realm of the empirical, but rests on *a priori* grounds. This paradoxically double quality with respect to the empirical allows aesthetic judgment to exist within a peculiar temporality: It both takes place in time while simultaneously generating a timeless rule retroactively employed to qualify the very act of judgment itself. The retrospective application of the rule is then said to condition the judgment. Further, and more importantly, this retroactive conditioning of the judgment provides the judge (him)self for the critique. This operation is explicitly stated to be (or begin) empirical because it must necessarily try out every object before it can assess that object's conformity to taste. In connection with the pleasure associated with aesthetic judgment, Kant writes:

---

17 Jacques Derrida, *The Truth in Painting*, trans. Geoff Bennington and Ian McLeod (Chicago and London: University of Chicago Press, 1987), 39.

> ... [T]he pleasure in a judgment of taste is indeed dependent on an empirical presentation and cannot be connected a priori with any concept (we cannot determine a priori what object will or will not conform to taste; *we must try it out* [man muß ihn versuchen]. (31, 102)

Aesthetic judgments are not made *a priori*. Rather, they rely on experience and experiment, and a remarkable harmony in the play of the faculties signals the finding of beauty. No determinable attribute of the object forms the basis of the judgment, Kant argues, though it supposes (in fact, ultimately demands) a subjective and universal assent among men[18] (30, 101). In this sense, the reflective quality of an aesthetic judgments is, in fact, double. It judges beauty (necessarily) in the absence of a concept and thereby generates a rule, thus also fulfilling the duty to search out the universal for a given particular with which the reflective judgment is charged. This generated rule, a product of reflection, is possessed of a remarkable productivity, that of constituting a universality of accord through the exemplary status of an aesthetic judgment.

The relationship between the imagination and the understanding in aesthetic judgments allows certain peculiarities of cognitive process to come to light. As Kant points out they provide the transcendental philosopher with a felicitous instance/insight:

> Diese besondere Bestimmung der Allgemeinheit eines ästhetischen Urteils, die sich in einem Geschmacksurteile antreffen läßt, ist eine Merkwürdigkeit, zwar nicht für den Logiker, aber wohl für den Transzendental-Philosophen, welche *seine* nicht geringe Bemühung auffordert, um den Ursprung derselben zu entdecken, dafür aber auch eine Eigenschaft unseres Erkenntnisvermögens aufdeckt, welche, ohne diese Zergliederung, unbekannt geblieben wäre. (127)

> This special [*besondere*] characteristic of an aesthetic judgment [of reflection], the universality [*Allgemeinheit*] to be found in judgments of taste, is a remarkable feature, not indeed for the logician but certainly for the transcendental

18 As Spivak argues, the condition of possibility of this subject of universal assent remains the foreclosure of other subjects' access to the position of narrator in the critique. Spivak, *A Critique of Postcolonial Reason*, 4-9. This ethico-political subject, Spivak further argues, presents the "only example of the concept of a natural yet rational being." (14) Spivak's argument marks the distinctions in Kant's *Critique of Judgment* between different forms of distancing in the name of the Kantian subject. "In fact in Kant, the 'uneducated' are specifically the child and the poor, the 'naturally uneducatable' is woman. By contrast, *der rohe Mensch*, man in the raw, can, in its signifying reach, accommodate the savage and the primitive." And in the corresponding footnote No. 20: "...the treatment of (the theme and figure of) woman is shown to be demonstrated abundantly by Kant's text, even if often in the ruse of disavowal. As I hope to show, the figure of the 'native informant' is, by contrast foreclosed. Rhetorically crucial at the most important moment in the argument, it is not part of the argument in any way. Was it in this rift that the seeds of the civilizing mission of today's universalist feminism were sown?" (13)

> philosopher. This universality requires a major effort on his part if he is to discover its origin, but it compensates him for this by revealing to him a property of our cognitive power which without this analysis would have remained unknown. (57)

Again, it is important to look at the original German to appreciate the play on *besonder/allgemein* that runs throughout the *Critique of Judgment*. As we can see, in forming a determinative judgment – the subsumption of a particular to a *given* concept – the imagination can be said to "work" for the understanding. In the case of a judgment of taste, however, one observes – indeed one *must* observe – the imagination at liberty. Kant writes:

> Wenn nun im Geschmacksurteile die Einbildungskraft in ihrer Freiheit betrachtet werden muß, so wird sie erstlich nicht reproduktiv, wie sie den Assoziationsgesetzen unterworfen ist, sondern als produktiv und selbsttätig (als *Urheberin* willkürlicher Formen möglicher Anschauungen) angenommen ... (160, emphasis mine)

> Therefore, in a judgment of taste the imagination must be considered in its freedom. This implies, first of all, that this power is here not taken as reproductive, where it is subject to the laws of association, but as productive and spontaneous (as the *originator* of chosen forms of possible intuitions). (91)

In the case of this autonomously productive activity of the imagination, one might say that the imagination is at liberty to "work for itself." It is the origin of *possible* intuitions by dint of composing arbitrary forms in accordance with its own laws and thus authors its own activity. The text moves quickly on, however, to assert that such conditions are contradictory; that the autonomy of the imagination is itself a contradiction.

> Allein daß die *Einbildungskraft frei* und doch von *selbst gesetzmäßig* sei, d.i. daß sie eine Autonomie bei sich führe, ist ein Widerspruch. Der Verstand allein gibt das Gesetz. (160)

> And yet, to say that the *imagination* is *free* and yet *lawful of itself*, i.e., that it carries autonomy with it, is a contradiction. The understanding alone gives the law. (91)

Looking closely at this exposition of the famous "autonomy of the imagination in aesthetic judgment" in Kant, one notices that the impossibility here averred is, in fact, overdetermined: the imagination is neither permitted this activity nor capable of it. Further, this disavowed im/possibility incorporates an awkward doubling in the German: "daß sie Autonomie bei sich führe" (*to run/lead/wield its own autonomy*) – the reflexive construction doubles the reflexivity already embedded in the term "autonomy." Mimicking the strange conditions in the gap or abyss in which the judgment operates, the imagination's contradictory autonomy introduces a simultaneously lawful and lawless scene of production. Nonetheless, the appearance of lawfulness thereby generated *must* be witnessed and assessed.[19]

The operation of reflective judgment is neither grounded on a concept in this process, nor does it provide one. In a sense, one might say that it is the medium of pure and experimentally directed "conceptuality." What aesthetic judgment reveals about judgment is that when it is reflective, the imagination, beyond its function of *applying* a priori concepts of the understanding, the sole law-giver, can become autonomously productive (and not merely reproductive) and thereby also provide an insight into the formation of concepts themselves (75). This productivity refers initially to the composition of arbitrary forms, but one could argue that it simultaneously produces the community of common aesthetic assent or at least makes a demand for the possibility of this community. Though not providing a concept, aesthetic judgment *produces a demand.* As such, the aesthetic could be construed to border here closely on the constitution of collectivities and the declarations of the political sphere.

Time and the Imagination

Already in its activity in the first *Critique* the operation of the imagination in the forging of the schematism had demonstrated an intimate relationship to the experience of time. It is the synthetic faculty of the imagination that connects appearances in succession, and thus causality is a concept of the understanding (not necessarily an attribute of things in themselves). Only by what precedes it does a given appearance acquire its time-relation, providing the ground for all experience. ("Principle of Sufficient Reason" – Second Analogy). Further, "Every transition in perception is a determination of time through the generation of this perception." (" ... I generate [erzeuge] time itself in the apprehension of the intuition."[20] It is our inner experience of time that provides the condition for judging causally. Thus, while the imagination ordinarily participates in the generation of time, in the case of judgment it introduces this temporal relation into practice. As Kant remarks: " ... the power of judgment cannot be taught but only practiced."[21]This thought heralds from an infinite regress of sorts that resem-

19 To what extent is the memory of the reader made responsible both for the initial positing of the imagination's autonomy and then charged with its negation? To what extent does that autonomy still play in the ear of the reader, once again facilitating the *Übergang* performed in the abyss?

20 Immanuel Kant, *Critique of Pure Reason*, trans. Paul Guyer (Cambridge, England: Cambridge University Press, 1998), 268.

21 Ibid., 267.

bles the regress that led the law of natural causality to reach its point of self-contradiction: Were there to be a rule on how to subsume under rules, that would again be a rule:

> Now if it [general logic] wanted to show generally how one ought to subsume under these rules, i.e., distinguish whether something stands under them or not, this could not happen except once again through a rule. But just because this is a rule, it would demand another instruction for the power judgment, and so it becomes clear that although the understanding is certainly capable of being instructed and equipped through rules, the power of judgment is a special [*besonderes*] talent that cannot be taught but only practiced.

In this sense, in the case of judgment, we witness a *specifically* empirical subject. While the synthesis always generates time, in the case of the judgment it also must come under the reign of that conditioning principle; not a given rule but an ongoing practice that points to a rule conditions the cultivation of judgment. One might say that already, by definition, it has a history. As Derrida has argued, the aesthetic judgment provides a concept of man outside of time while also conditioning this being historically.

> The exemplary (*exemplarisch*) is a singular product (*Produkt*) – since it is an example which is immediately valid for all. Only certain exemplary products can have this effect of quasi-rules. Whence the historical, cultural, pragmatico-anthropological character of taste, which is constituted after the event [après coup], after the production, by means of example. The absence of concept thus liberates this horizon of historical productivity. But this historicity is that of an exemplar which gives itself as an example only to the extent that it signals, empirically, toward a structural and universal principle of accord, which is absolutely ahistorical.[22]

With a kind of slip stitch, the necessarily empirical *Versuch* of any single aesthetic judgment possesses a double temporality: it transpires in time while still participating in the ahistorical universality of accord it brings to light. From this vantage, it either reveals this accord, or, were one to entertain the possibility, it demands that such an accord *come into being*. The unexpectedly radical productivity of what should 'simply' serve a reproductive function thus either presents a structural universality among men or it produces it.

In this differential, the connection between the asymmetrically related pieces of the critique finds its movement, for, with the liberation of "this horizon of historical productivity," Kant's aesthetic judgment also reveals for us something of the project to be undertaken in the second half of the

---

22 Derrida, *The Truth in Painting*, 109.

third *Critique*, the "Critique of Teleological Judgment." In the aesthetic portion of the critique, we are instructed in the unique ability of the reflective judgment to *observe* objects in their formal finality without assigning to them an end/purpose (*Zweck*).

> Also können wir eine Zweckmäßigkeit der Form nach, auch ohne daß wir ihr einen Zweck (als die Materie des nexus finalis) zum Grunde legen, wenigstens beobachten, und an Gegenständen, wiewohl nicht anders als durch Reflexion, bemerken. (135)

> Hence we can at least observe a purposiveness as to form and take note of it in objects – even if only by reflection – without basing it on a purpose (as the matter of the *nexus finalis*). (65)

Here we have an exposition of precisely that capability betrayed by the aesthetic judgment, which will later be put to use in the teleological judgment. Insofar as it legislates only to itself – and the imagination in this capacity is capable of the generation of arbitrary forms – reflective judgment becomes a kind of virtual mechanism that can unite the peculiar capacity of aesthetic observation with the testing of hypotheses. "Observing teleologically" (without assigning specific concepts) renders the speculative zone of heuristic observation Kant proposes, and reflection facilitates experimental testing in the indeterminate terrain and errant jurisdiction of the judgment.

Though no single clarification may be taken for granted when reading the third *Critique*, Kant does make the following clear statement concerning the relationship between natural ends and natural beauty:

> ... [S]o legen wir ihr doch hiedurch gleichsam eine Rücksicht auf unser Erkenntnisvermögen nach der Analogie eines Zwecks bei; und so können wir die *Naturschönheit* als *Darstellung* des Begriffs der formalen (bloß subjektiven), und die *Naturzwecke* als Darstellung des Begriffs einer realen (objektiven) Zweckmäßigkeit ansehen, deren eine wir durch Geschmack (ästhetisch, vermittelst des Gefühls der Lust), die andere durch Verstand und Vernunft (logisch, nach Begriffen) beurteilen. (104)

> ...we are still attributing to nature, on the analogy of a purpose, a concern, as it were, for our cognitive power. Hence we may regard *natural beauty* as the *exhibition* of the concept of formal (merely subjective) purposiveness, and may regard *natural purposes* as the exhibition of the concept of a real (objective) purposiveness, the first of which we judge by taste (aesthetically, by means of the feeling of pleasure), and the second by understanding and reason (logically, according to concepts). (33)

Though the consideration of natural ends is here aligned with the objective and concept-driven, it is important to recall that teleological judgment has only been provisionally annexed to the critique of judgment "in the case of certain natural objects" (36). Moreover, it finds itself circumstantially displaced from the realm of pure reason (and doctrine) to be deployed in test-cognitions whose subjective and formal determinations border very closely on the determination of the practical will through freedom. The models and conclusions generated in these tests are not binding, though they may also, like aesthetic judgments, become exemplary. To recall Kant's own description of the exemplary status of aesthetic judgment:

> Rather, as a necessity that is thought in an aesthetic judgment, it can only be called *exemplary*, i.e., a necessity of the assent of *everyone* to a judgment that is regarded as an example of a universal rule that we are unable to state. (85)

In keeping with an overarching enlightenment ideal, the empty placeholder of aesthetic judgment's example (a universal rule we cannot state) houses a potential universality – to this extent aesthetic judgment points to a possible future in historical being and Kant's figure of the *Naturzweck* carries this indication further.

Ein Naturzweck (A Natural Purpose)

At the end of the eighteenth century in European natural science, a search was underway for a simple set of laws governing the sphere of biological growth and reproduction that could match Newton's laws in the area of physics.[23] The second half of the final volume of Kant's critical philosophy, "Critique Of Teleological Judgment" devotes itself to the possibility of such a systematic unity behind the laws governing natural growth and individual/species reproduction, and his critique offers counsel as to the justifiable use of teleological judgment in natural research (*Naturforschung*).[24]

---

23 On the genesis of the term "biology" Timothy Lenoir explains: "Eventually the term 'biology' proposed originally by Jean Baptiste Lamarck and Gotthelf Reinhold Treviranus in 1802, came to identify the discipline whose object was to be 'the different forms and phenomena of life, the conditions and laws of their existence as well as the causes that determine them." Timothy Lenoir, *The Strategy of Life: Teleology and Mechanic in 19th Century Biology* (Boston: D. Reidel Publishing Company, 1982), 1. In *Das Ende der Naturgeschichte,* Wolf Lepenies gives an historical example of how quickly the concept proliferated. "Wie schnell der Begriff 'Biologie' sich durchsetzt, zeigt sich an Carl Gustav Carus, der im Jahre 1811 zum Gegenstand seiner Dissertation nichts geringeres als den Entwurf einer allgemeinen Lebenslehre, *Specimen Biologiae generalis*, wählen kann" Wolf Lepenies, *Das Ende der Naturgeschichte* (Vienna: Hanser Verlag, 1976), 30.

24 See Barbara Stollberg-Rilinger, *Europa im Jahrhundert der Aufklärung* (Stuttgart: Reclam, 2000) for a helpful introduction to the rise of the new life sciences. Stollinger argues that this search for first principles was also consonant with the eighteenth-century goal of overcoming dualisms inherited from seventeenth century Rationalism and thereby bringing nature

As historian of science, Timothy Lenoir, points out, while Kant did not set the program for research, he spoke to the late eighteenth century scientists' struggle to "establish a foundation for constructing a consistent body of unified theory for the life sciences which could adapt the methods and conceptual framework of Newtonian science to the special requirements of investigating biological organisms."[25] As Kant puts it in the third *Critique*, we "rejoice" and in fact are "relieved of a want" (representing a minor incursion into the sphere of disinterestedness) when we discover systematic unity behind "merely empirical laws."[26]

The definition of the *Naturzweck* in the third *Critique* surpassed the vitalism vs. mechanism distinction by helping to pose questions regarding the "causal relations of organic form and function."[27] Defined only in terms of concepts provided by the reflective judgment, the *Naturzweck* offered a model of the organism as teleologically self-determining. In doing so it drew on the work of Johannes Fr. Blumenbach (1752-1848) in *Über den Bildungstrieb (Nisus fomativus) und seinen Einfluss auf die Generation und Reproduction* (1781).[28] Blumenbach's published observations on the regenerative capacity of organic matter enter the third *Critique* in an appendix (and on a structural level) as the figure of an epistemological problem. His theory of a formative drive in living matter (*Bildungstrieb*) offers a crucial bridge (as exemplar) to the unique organization of a *Naturzweck* in Kant's definition. It may well have a bearing on the coherence of the third *Critique* itself, since Blumenbach's speculative *Bildungstrieb* triggers a series of

---

and reason into proximity. "Newtons Himmelsmechanik übte auch deshalb eine so große Faszination auf das Denken des 18. Jahrhunderts aus, weil sie die rationalistische Trennung von Geist und Materie ignorierte. ... Damit führte er eindrucksvoll vor Augen, dass es metaphysischer Spekulation überhaupt nicht bedurfte, um ein funktionierendes, richtige Voraussagen erzeugendes und experimentell überprüfbares Modell der Welt aufzustellen" (173).

25 Lenoir, *Strategy of Life,* 2. Cassirer points out that Kant's reception has often lost track of the primary interest of the "Critique of Teleological Judgment" – the question of metaphysical teleology – by focusing too much on the comparison between Kant and Darwin from the vantage of more recent scientific knowledge. Cassirer, *Kant's Life,* 283-284.

26 The whole passage runs: ". . .daher wir auch, gleich als ob es ein glücklicher unsre Absicht begünstigender Zufall wäre, erfreuet (eigentlich eines Bedürfnisses entledigt) werden, wenn wir eine solche systematische Einheit unter bloß empirischen Gesetzen antreffen . . ." (93). "This is also why we rejoice (actually we are relieved of a need) when, just as if it were a lucky chance favoring our aim, we do find such systematic unity among merely empirical laws" (23-24).

27 For the importance of Kant's readings in the natural sciences and the relevance of his activity as a reviewer, see Karl J. Fink, "Kant's Concept of Telos: Reviews Shaping Anthropology," in *The Eighteenth Century German Book Review*, ed. Herbert Rowland and KarlJ. Fink (Heidelberg: Universitätsverlag, 1995), 169-180.

28 Johann Friedrich Blumenbach, *Über den Bildungstrieb* (Göttingen: 1781).

causal conundra for Kant's critique which prove remarkably useful in facilitating the forward motion of the exposition.

In the example of the tree offered in §64 *Von dem Eigentümlichen Charakter der Dinge als Naturzwecke*, the point is made that, in reproducing itself, the tree not only produces another tree ("zeugt erstlich einen andern Baum") but also a species: for itself *and* for another.[29] (318, 249) Further, when viewed as a system, the plant appears to be possessed of a motive force that does not reside *outside* of "what it is." Kant remarks that one is pushed toward the "*uneigentlich*" expression of matter *as related to itself* as organizational force. Like the imagination, it possesses from this standpoint a contradictory autonomy: a tree, as *Naturzweck*, actively generates both the *form* of its individuality and its generality, and in this sense it mediates between universal and particular in a way that is instructive for the third *Critique*. It *appears* as if the causality observed in the natural purpose had come about through a causality only reason can have, that is, to act according to purposes in accordance with *Vorstellungen* such as a will would (248, 317).

> We said in the preceding section that if a thing is a natural product but yet we are to cognize it as possible only as a natural purpose, then it must have this character: it must relate to itself in such a way that it is both cause and effect of itself. But this description is not quite appropriate [*uneigentlich*: not literal, figurative] and determinate and still needs to be derived from a determinate concept. (251) [§65]

The recourse to a catachrestic use of language to introduce an entity reciprocally related to itself as both cause and effect both motivates the search for a new form of lawfulness and clearly mirrors the questions central to a critique of judgment. These objects do not solely present to human apprehension a *nexus effectivus* (wherein a series of effects produces causes in an exclusively forward motion) but a *nexus finalis* (wherein each effect can

29 On examples in Kant, see Cathy Caruth, "The Force of Example" in *Empirical Truths and Critical Fictions: Locke, Wordsworth, Kant, Freud* (Baltimore: Johns Hopkins University Press, 1991). On a passage from the *Metaphysical Foundations of Natural Science,* in which Kant reflects on the recourse taken by metaphysics to derive its pure concepts from "the general doctrine of body" Caruth remarks: "What surprises Kant, however, is not just the dependence of the 'form' on any illustrative 'intuition,' but rather the dependence of the form specifically on '*external* intuition' or the 'general doctrine of body.' External intuition, here, is not just a content that gives meaning to the conceptual form, but itself has a 'form' and 'principles' in the science of dynamics: it is another 'form' which is the meaning of the 'mere form' of thought. The need for something 'external' to thought is thus, here, different from the need for 'experience' in general which Kant emphasizes throughout the first *Critique*: it is another kind of externality represented by the dependence of the form of transcendental philosophy on the form of Newtonian science, a doubling of form and form" (65).

also be construed as the cause of what caused it), and the appearance of this latter form of causality forms the crux of the operative "Antinomy of Judgment" which introduces the teleological model.

Just as Kant suggests in the second introduction that judgment, like reason and understanding, must be possessed of its own special principle, in the second section of the third *Critique*, judgment also acquires its own antinomy. Antinomies present impasses or blockages that render the movement of critique possible. They result from the confrontation of two conflicting, but wholly tenable, concepts of reason and are motivated dialectically. As Kant asserts, determinative judgment runs no risk of confronting an antinomy because it lacks autonomy: it merely subsumes particulars under principles, but does not itself generate principles (§69). The reflective judgment, however, runs this risk because of its autonomous progress *toward* an unknown law. For laws not yet given, reflective judgment must employ concepts *potentially*, generate its own nondeterminative/subjective maxims, and *possibly* experience a conflict between heterogeneous laws.

In the case of the "Antinomy of Judgment," the two conflicting maxims are as follows: first, "all production of material things and their forms must be judged to be possible in terms of mechanistic laws," and second, "some products of material nature cannot be judged to be possible in terms of merely mechanical laws (judging them requires a quite different causal law – viz., that of final causes)."[30] The antinomy requires that in default of a mechanical explanation – and where an alternate mode of causality presents itself to our understanding – teleological judgment, in its reflective character, be engaged. In the space opened up by this antinomy – a virtual vista liberated by its impasse – a project of natural science takes shape that concedes the transcendent character of the ultimate and necessary union of mechanical and teleological principles in the same products of nature (297, 367). The heterogeneous principle of the organized being cannot be regarded as anything but founded in the supersensible and cannot be determinate. The project of *investigating* its features thus grapples with the enigma of apparently divergent causal forces and must consider the possibility of a distinct life force in nature to which mechanical causes would be subordinate. While no resort can be made to other than mecha-

30 Kant, *Critique of Judgment*, 267. "Die erste Maxime derselben ist der Satz: Alle Erzeugung materieller Dinge und ihrer Formen muß, als nach bloß mechanischen Gesetzen möglich, beurteilt werden." And "Die zweite Maxime ist der Gegensatz: Einige Produkte der materiellen Natur können nicht, als nach bloß mechanischen Gesetzen möglich, beurteilt werden (ihre Beurteilung erfordert ein ganz anderes Gesetz der Kausalität, nämlich das der Endursachen" (336).

nistic explanations of natural phenomena, the paucity of these explanations, the relative insufficiency of their insight into the true workings of natural products, demands an openness in the work of observation.

The double necessity of the peculiarity and limitation of human cognition, on the one hand, and the insufficiency of mechanistic models of explanation, on the other, enter into a productive bind. Though, as Kant states in the above-cited paragraph from the appendix, "Methodology of Teleological Judgment," "every effort must be made to discover the mechanism subordinate to any particular purpose in nature." The uncertainty involved in this project opens up room for conjecture concerning a possible biological force to match the force of gravity.[31] Kant concludes this paragraph with reference to Blumenbach's *Bildungstrieb*:

> ... Yet by appealing to this principle of an original organization, a principle that is inscrutable to us, he [Herr Hofr. Blumenbach] leaves an indeterminable and yet unmistakable share to natural mechanism. The ability of the matter in an organized body to [take on] this organization he calls a formative impulse. (It is distinguished from the merely mechanical formative force that all matter has, [but] stands under the higher guidance and direction, as it were, of that formative force.) (311)

The transfer of the word *Vermögen* (power, ability) to matter itself bears notice. It is precisely the inextricability of the form of the matter and that matter itself, the possibility that matter is self-forming, doubly present to itself as effect and cause (reflexively self-generating?), that motivates the questions brought together here regarding organized beings.

The organized being ("organisiertes Wesen" generally translated as "organism" in English) is neither machine, as a materialist of Julien Offray de La Mettrie's order would consider, nor is it fully understood and explained through laws of motion. The organized being produces its own food or energy source and in this activity is more than a clock in that it produces, consumes, and reproduces itself. What for human understanding can only be thought of as a *Technik der Natur* (technique of nature) exists in Kant's terminology in apposition to a *produktives Vermögen* (productive capacity). Not inert matter in motion but matter as productive

---

31 In the introduction to his translation of Kant's *Critique of Judgment*, Werner Pluhar stresses the fact that this admonition to search for further mechanistic explanations to subordinate to particular purposes in nature not be understood as the dissolution of the antinomy of reason (discussed above), which necessitates the critique of teleological judgment (xcix-c). That antinomy has different consequences for the coherence of the whole body of the Kantian critiques and for the program in naturalist research which Kant suggests. Hannah Ginsborg has presented arguments as to why a mechanical explanation will not suffice: Hannah Ginsborg, "Two Kinds of Mechanical Inexplicability in Kant and Aristotle," *Journal of the History of Philosophy* 42 (1): 33-65.

capacity: the wheels and cogs of a time piece may move in concert, but they do not produce, consume, reproduce, or heal themselves.[32] While this distinction may seem obviously "biological" to a modern reader, Kant walks a thin line in eighteenth century naturalism, between vitalism and mechanism.[33] The presence of Blumenbach's research is quite pronounced in this illustrative digression for, though here unnamed, it is clearly Blumenbach's green polyp that stands across from the vestigal example of the clock as image of nature's mechanism.

> Generation und Reproduction – Zeugung und diese Wiederersetzung, sind beides Modificationen *ein und eben derselben Kraft*: die letztre ist nicht anders, als eine partielle Wiederholung der erstern: und ein Licht über die eine von beiden verbreitet, muß sicher auch die andre zugleich aufhellen. (emphasis mine)

> Generation and reproduction – procreation and this restoring of lost parts are both modifications of one and the same force: the latter is not other than a partial repetition of the first, and a light cast on one must certainly illumine the other.[34]

Research into the regenerative capacity of the polyp represented an intervention in the preformation vs. epigenesis debate on reproduction.[35] The

---

32 Hannah Ginsborg has argued that the problem of finding mechanical laws by which to explain organisms does not lie so much with their difference from machines such as clocks but in that "they possess a regular structure, and display regularities in functioning, which cannot be accounted for in terms of the basic physical and chemical powers of matter alone." Hannah Ginsborg, "Kant's Biological Teleology and Its Philosophical Significance," in *Blackwell Companion to Kant*, ed. Graham Bird (Oxford: Blackwell Publishing, 2006), 455-69.

33 For a discussion of this "line," see Lenoir, *The Strategy of Life*, chapter 1 "Vital Materialism: Blumenbach, Kant and the Teleomechanical Approach to Life." Lenoir argues that Blumenbach wanted to avoid treating biological organization as a result of the superimposition of a separate force, *Lebenskraft*, or soul on inorganic matter, attempting thereby to avoid both mechanical reductionism and vitalism; an attempt that results in the postulation of the "immanent teleological character of this vital force" (20). Lenoir goes on to assert: "Kant was quick to seize upon the *Bildungstrieb* as exemplifying exactly what he intended by a 'regulative principle' in theory construction" (22). See also Helmut Müller-Sievers, *Self-Generation: Biology, Philosophy and Literature around 1800* (Palo Alto: Stanford University Press, 1997), 6. "Kant and the early epigenist researchers at the University of Göttingen knew well that epigenesis is a transcendental concept in precisely this 'mechanical' sense: we assume it because all other assumptions come at too high a cost."

34 Reese translation.

35 Again, see Lenoir and Müller-Sievers for a refined treatment of these positions. Simply stated: epigenesis names the hypothesis of a development involving the gradual diversification and differentiation of an initially undifferentiated entity; preformation names the now discredited theory in biology that every germ cell contains the organism of its kind fully formed and complete in all its parts and that development consists merely in increase in size from microscopic proportions to those of the adult. An example of this idea can be

reconstitution of injured parts Blumenbach observes in the polyp is understood as a "fulfilling" of the form which defines the whole. Thus reconstitution becomes a kind of repetition of reproduction. In both instances, the matter itself provides the form. Blumenbach characterizes the *Bildungstrieb*'s participation in the growth of the organism with the verb "*beiwohnen*" (in-dwelling) in this passage but he elaborates in a later passage the necessity to remain circumspect with regard to its cause.[36]

> Hoffentlich ist für die mehresten Leser die Erinnerung sehr überflüssig, daß das Wort Bildungstrieb, so gut wie die Worte Attraction, Schwere etc. zu nichts mehr und nichts weniger dienen soll, als eine Kraft zu bezeichnen, deren constante Wirkung aus der Erfahrung anerkannt worden, deren Ursache aber so gut wie die Ursache der genannten, noch so allgemein anerkannten Naturkräfte für uns qualitas occulta ist. (25-26)

> Hopefully it is unnecessary to remind most readers that the word *Bildungstrieb*, as wel as the words attraction, weight, etc. serve no more and no less to designate a force whose constant action has been recognized, [but] whose cause, just as much as the cause of the other generally recognized natural forces, is for us *qualitas occulta*.[37]

Blumenbach, later to become a careful reader of Kant, resists "determining," to use the Kantian vocabulary, the *Bildungstrieb*. He does not posit it as a substance nor attempt to adduce its cause, but undertakes to observe it in terms of a teleological form of causality.[38] The conservation of form reveals itself to observation, but does not undo its mystery. Nonetheless, Blumenbach's research introduces the possibility to his reader that *all* of

---

found in Sterne's *Tristram Shandy*'s homonculous. Sterne's novel already points to the potential for political satire by vesting the homonculous with the rights and claims of humanity. Laurence Sterne, *Tristram Shandy* (New York: W. W. Norton & Company, 1980), 2.

36 Blumenbach's definition of the "*Trieb*" runs as follows: "Ein Trieb, der folglich zu den Lebenskräften gehört, der aber eben so deutlich von den übrigen Arten der Lebenskraft der organisirten Körper (der Contractilität, Irritibilität, Sensibilität etc.) als von den allgemeinen physischen Kräften der Körper überhaupt, verschieden ist; der die erste wichtigste Kraft zu aller Zeugung, Ernäherung, und Reproduction zu seyn scheint, und den man um ihn von andern Lebenskräften zu unterscheiden, mit dem Namen des Bildungstriebes (nisus formatiuus) bezeichnen kann" (24-25).

37 Reese translation.

38 See Eckart Förster for a fascinating discussion of *intellektuelle Anschauung* versus *intuitiver Verstand* and the possibility the the former need not be considered the first origin ("Weltursache") but rather "als a) produktive Einheit von Möglichkeit (Denken) und Wirklichkeit (Sein), und b) als nichtsinnliche Anschauung von Dinge an sich." (179) Eckart Förster, "Die Bedeutung von §§76,77 von Kant's *Kritik der Urteilskraft* für die Entwicklung der nachkantischen Philosophie," *Zeitschrift für Philosophische Forschung*, Band 56 (2002), 2. Förster's essay also argues that Goethe construed Kant's argument concerning teleological observation as presenting the possibility of observing an organism *in its temporal development*, but wherein each stage would be comprehended simultaneously.

the material constituent of a particular natural purpose is informed by the drive to complete that formation. The imprint of the whole thus spans and coordinates all separate parts and seems to point to a force of life at work *in* matter. The evidence of this suffusion of matter with a formative drive, meanwhile, remains a puzzle of incommensurable forms of causation.

Blumenbach's *qualita occultas* thus contributes to an enabling antinomy for Kantian critique. In §73 "None of the Above Systems Accomplishes What It Alleges to Accomplish" [*Keines Der Obigen Systeme Leistet Das Was Es Vorgibt*], the concept of "living matter" ultimately represents the false promise of circular reasoning.

> And yet we cannot even think of living matter as possible. (The [very] concept of it involves a contradiction, since the essential character of matter is lifelessness, [in Latin] *inertia.*
>
> But this means that our explanation can only move in a circle: we try to derive the natural purposiveness in organized beings from the life of matter, while yet we are familiar with this life only in organized beings and hence cannot form a concept of the possibility of this purposiveness unless we have experienced such beings.[39] (276, 345-346)

The dilemma of causation cannot be resolved through the mere assertion of life, and the close of the "Critique of Teleological Judgment" contains pessimistic pronouncements concerning the rise of a "Newton of biology" or the possibility of ever bringing all the phenomena of nature under the scope of mechanical laws (373). Indeed, one of the most difficult challenges for the interpretation of the elaborate structure of *Critique of Judgment* concerns the status of teleological judgment by the work's end.

Kant's argument oscillates between a round refusal of the capacity for human cognition to reconcile mechanical and teleological principles and a barely suggested possibility that judgment's special principle of the purposiveness of nature could allow, through teleological observation, a fortunate discovery of greater and greater levels of generality in the investigation of the laws of nature. In the appendix, Kant clearly states that he refuses to posit "objectively purposive forms of matter" as do those who assert the "ontological concept of a simple substance." He argues against

39 Pluhar provides the following footnote attached to "life" in this passage: "In the *Critique of Practical Reason* (Ak. V, 9n), *life* is defined (narrowly) as "the ability of a being to act according to laws of the power of desire." In the *Metaphysics of Morals* (Ak. IV, 211), Kant defines it similarly as "the ability of a being to act in conformity with its presentations" (276). Though the definition of life will come forward in Kant's *oeuvre* in various articulations, the consistent thread throughout is a capacity for action on the part of a desiring subject. In the third *Critique* this desiring agency is linked directly with the susperrsensible freedom, therefore pointing to a specifically moral form of agency.

this position, which he attributes to the pantheists, that it can still not be proven how this substance relates to itself as its own purpose.[40] (§80, 307) His critique is thus clearly less prepared to attribute an objective *Bildungstrieb* to mere matter and his argument focuses much more decisively on the discussion of the limits of human understanding and the manner in which they negatively outline the possibility of an alternate form of understanding for which the causalities of freedom and nature would not be incommensurate. For this discussion, the recommendation made to the sciences to proceed reflectively with teleological observation would seem to be incidental to the true project of the third *Critique*. Though the desire to pass from critique to natural science is clearly evinced in works such as *Metaphysische Anfangsgründe der Naturwissenschaft*, and Kant's dilation on natural form must be regarded as profoundly inspired by the research of his day, the final passages of "Critique of Teleological Judgment" clearly demonstrate a strong commitment to maintaining the problem posed by the antinomy of judgment. What is the sense, then, of securing the conjectures of reflective judgment for teleology? As Kant is not only interested in delineating impossibility but also in sketching counterpossibilities along its contour, there ought to be some productive dimension to the teleological experiment.

A Critical Passage into History

The indefinite terrain of reflective judgment, in this case concerned with the products of nature (akin to the theoretical), simultaneously mirrors the practical. The conjectures undertaken concerning the possible teleological organization of those natural products termed *Naturzwecke,* like the moral command and the judgment of taste, are prescriptive and not descriptive (regulative, not determinative). Though Kant's text insists that the teleological analogy cannot explain (*erklären*) but only describe, it simultaneously terms these descriptions *regulative*. The potential commensuration of accidental mechanical laws with a necessary finality of matter/form parallels, at least on a systematic level, the practical nature of moral laws as commands. That is to say, when in the case of moral commands, "reason expresses this necessity, not by an 'is' or 'happens' (being or fact), but by an 'ought to be,'" it responds to the peculiar human condition of differentiating between the possible and the actual and the attendant incommensurability of the theoretical and the practical. (*Critique of Judgment*, §76, 287) The regulative principle of this duty "does not objectively determine

40 For an illuminating discussion of Kant's *Critique of Judgment* in the context of the pantheist controversy see Zammito, *The Genesis of Kant's Critique of Judgment*, 228-247.

the character of freedom as a form of causality." Instead, it makes "the rule [that we ought] to act according to that idea into a command for everyone" (287). Now, while one cannot properly construe the peculiar form of the *Naturzweck* as a command, it remains, in Kant's exposition, a necessity for human cognition and, therefore, a subjectively universal, regulative principle. Further, the unavoidable differentiation between a natural mechanism and a natural purpose constitutes a unique predilection of human understanding. Unable to subsume the particulars in question under a given universal, the relationship between reason and understanding generates the spheres of possibility and actuality according to which human cognition operates. The contingency of sensuous human cognition can relate to the contingency of any given particular only in terms of finality, but that finality, in turn, can only be regulative.

In §64, the issue of "will" plagues the initial discussion. A will would by definition need to be at work if things were to be presented (*vorgestellt*) as "acting according to purposes" (*nach Zwecken zu handeln*) (317). The apparent conformity to a concept of reason of the contingent form of the natural product gives rise to the cognitive presentation (*Vorstellung*) of the object as possible only as a purpose/end. Kant passes immediately from these remarks on the apparent activity of a will in the formation of the natural purpose to a discussion of geometrical figures. In a brief interlude, Kant imagines the event of discovering a regular hexagon drawn in the sands of apparently uninhabited land. The reasoning source of causation that would appear to be evidenced by this geometrical figure causes its perceiver to assume its provenance as other than ". . . the sand, the neighboring sea, the wind or animals with their footprints . . ." *(der Sand, das benachbarte Meer, die Winde, oder auch Tiere mit ihren Fußtritten)* (317, Reese translation). The trace left on the sand is not necessarily a sign or message, but it does bespeak a conceptual source of production. It introduces an eerie strain into the empty presence of pure nature.

The description recalls the scenario of an encounter of exploration reminiscent of *Robinson Crusoe*: as if a solitary will stumbled across the sign of another presence. In the designation of human cognition as fundamentally predicated on the distinction between actual and possible, a fictive realm emerges which brings *Critique of Judgment* closer in some elements of its exposition to the speculative fictions of 18th-century language-origin theories than the other two critiques. The thought of a divine intelligence is often present in Kant's consideration of human cognitive faculties in the guise of an alien being with superior/different powers of intuition.[41]

---

41 In the case of the second half of the third *Critique*, this figure is that of the intuitive understanding that can legislate the particular as well as the universal. Pluhar sums up the situa-

Not footprints but what appear to be traces are discovered throughout nature and the potential of their significatory value – both within the mere fact of their existence and the possibility of what they reproduce – presents an important challenge to the critique (though again, they refer only to the peculiarities of our own powers of cognition and do not betray things in themselves).[42] "Life-forms" themselves appear as challenging evidence of the potential of another presence: and it is noteworthy that they, in turn, double themselves in that they are simultaneously conceived of as possessing the appearance of products of technical activity and as productive forces. Though organisms (*Naturzwecke*) in Kant's definition are not construed as messages any more than the hexagon discovered in the sands of a deserted beach, the task they present to human understanding introduces the uncanny, fragmentary glimpse of an intuition wherein incommensurable forms of finality could become commensurate.

The phenomenon of growth and organization in *Naturzwecke* disturbs the boundary of the matter/idea divide in ways exemplary for questions concerning the activity of judgment. As was the case in the critique of aesthetic judgment, issues and parallels to the will insinuate themselves. In the *Metaphysical Foundations of Natural Science* (1786), Kant defines life as "the capacity of a substance to determine itself to act from an internal principle" in contradistinction to the "lifelessness" of inertial matter. (Leben *heißt das Vermögen einer* Substanz, *sich aus einem* inneren Prinzip *zum Handeln*...) He hastens, however, to add that "we know of no other principle of a substance to change its state but desire." (*Nun kennen wir kein*

---

tion thus: "The concept of the supersensible basis of nature's purposiveness is the concept of an intuitive understanding with its intellectual intuition; but our understanding, unable to think the concept of an intuitive understanding, instead thinks of the supersensible basis of nature's purposiveness as an intelligent cause of the world in terms of purposes" (ci). In Heidegger's reading of Kant, this kind of intuition is described as "creative intuition." (Heidegger, *Kant and the Problem of Metaphysics*, 25). Again, see Förster, "Die Bedeutung," for a reading which distinguishes between intuitive understanding and intellectual intuition and which would not *necessarily* land the *Critique's* reader in theology.

42 See *The Truth in Painting* for the discussion of another scene of discovery in the aesthetic section of the third *Critique*. In the footnote that closes the Third Moment of the critique of aesthetic judgment, Kant takes the discovery of a handle-less stone tool unearthed from a burial site as an illustration of the difference between a tool and a work of art. The mutilated finality of the incomplete tool is not to be judged beautiful as in the case of the illusive finality of the tulip. (Derrida, *The Truth in Painting*, 83-101). In the instance of the geometrical figure discussed above, another scene of discovery supplements the exposition of the critique, but in this case the suggestiveness of its discovering evidence links it to an uncanny presence of life, rather than to an aura of death. The freedom of the flower's finality, which raises it above the tool, is inverted in the second scene in which nature's "freedom" from the laws of human cognition (Kant will indeed express nature's independence in these terms) moves closer and closer to moral freedom's necessity.

anderes inneres Prinzip einer Substanz, ihren Zustand zu verändern, als das Begehren...)[43]

The peculiar character of the *Naturzweck* does not solely provide a better description of natural things than the mechanistic analogy to the clock: it challenges the exercise of judgment. The organized and self-organizing being presents to our consideration a "formative force that propagates itself." This force deflates the analogy to art, which as Kant remarks, is "too little said," and if anything introduces paradoxes of causation and maddening doubles as in his subsequent remark: "Näher tritt man vielleicht dieser unerforschlichen Eigenschaft, wenn man sie ein Analogon des Lebens nennt" (323). ("We might be closer if we call this inscrutable property of nature an *analogue of life*") (254). Not an analogue of art, but an analogue of life, of "the capacity of a substance to determine itself to act from an internal principle." One must guard against falling into the fallacy of hylozoism and also resist the temptation of deferring the problem by invoking the agency of a soul. For this reason, at this impasse, the natural purpose performs the invaluable service of presenting a limit to understanding: "Genau zu reden hat also die Organisation der Natur nichts Analogisches mit irgend einer Kausalität, die wir kennen" (323). *(Strictly speaking, therefore, the organization of nature has nothing analogous to any causality known to us)* (254). It also offers a radical rupture in causal thinking and introduces a highly specific conceptualization of self-organization and self-reference to the repertoire of part-to-whole models or modalities.

Kant's carefully wrought exposition of the self-organized and self-organizing can be considered with respect to at least two consequences. The first, as mentioned above, is the recommendation it makes to the natural sciences – to hold out, as it were, for a keener understanding of motive life force. The second, though, will prove to be its relation to political and cultural life.

Final End of Nature (*Letzter Zweck der Natur*)

Kant offers a description of the predominance of forces of destruction in nature with a grim lyricism that highlights not the work of purpose in nature but the violence of natural process.

> Land and sea contain memorials of mighty devastations that long ago befell them and all creatures living on or in them. Indeed, their entire structure, the

43 Immanuel Kant, *Schriften zur Naturphilosophie,* Hrsg. von Wilhelm Weischedel (Frankfurt a.M.: Suhrkamp, 1968), 109-110. Immanuel Kant, *Metaphysical Foundations of Natural Sciene,* trans. James W. Ellington, in *Immanuel Kant: Philosophy of Material Nature* (Indianapolis: Hackett Publishing, 1985), 105-106.

> strata of the land and the boundaries of the sea, look quite like the product of savage, all-powerful forces of a nature working in a state of chaos. The shape of the land, its structure and its slope, may now seem very purposively arranged: to receive water from the air, to feed the water veins between diverse kinds of layers of soil (each [suitable] for all sorts of products), and to direct the rivers. But a closer investigation of them proves that they are in fact merely the result of eruptions, either of fire or of water, or of upheavals of the ocean. (315)

The appearance of a hexagon drawn in such sands might appear too fragile to face these massive movements of destruction unless we recall the refusal in the earlier exposition of the "sublime" to grant material force an edge against the infinity of reason.

> Wir haben im Vorigen gezeigt, daß wir den Menschen nicht bloß, wie alle organisierte Wesen, als Naturzweck, sondern auch hier auf Erden als den letzten Zweck der Natur, in Beziehung auf welchen alle übrige Naturdinge ein System von Zwecken ausmachen, nach Grundsätzen der Vernunft, zwar nicht für die bestimmende, doch für die reflektierende Urteilskraft, zu beurteilen hinreichende Ursache haben. (387)

> We have shown in the preceding section that [certain] principles of reason give us sufficient grounds for judging man – though reflectively rather than determinately – to be not merely a natural purpose, which we may judge all organized beings to be, but also to be the ultimate purpose by reference to which all other natural things constitute a system of purposes. (317)

In reflective judgment we have sufficient cause to judge man to be not only "Naturzweck" but also "letzter Zweck der Natur." This assessment balances precariously on a dizzying formal structure in which ends are mirrored in the proposing of ends – a kind of split-level infinite regress:

> Man is indeed the only being on earth that has understanding and hence an ability to set himself purposes of his own choice, and in this respect he holds the title of lord of nature; and if we regard nature as a teleological system, then it is man's vocation to be the ultimate purpose of nature, but always subject to a condition: he must have the understanding and *the will to give* both nature and himself reference to a purpose that can be independent of nature, self-sufficient, and a final purpose. The final purpose, however, we must not seek within nature at all. (318, emphasis mine)

As the setter of ends, man sets himself up as the end, and rendered in the subjunctive mood, this setting-oneself-ends-as-end predicates itself on an act of will and constitutes a giving of reference (*Zweckbeziehung zu geben*). The condition placed on the reign of man is precisely that he give himself such a relation to ends, that he refer himself to them, independently of nature. Here the paradox of history comes into play, because only through its self-sufficiency, its independence from nature, does this activity of setting ends make of man a final purpose, though this "must not be sought in nature." The end of nature is now outside of it. In Gilles Deleuze's very lucid summary:

> In so far as the last end is nothing other than the final end, it is the object of a fundamental paradox: the last end of sensible nature is an end that this nature itself is not sufficient to realize (CJ para. 84) [§84 is cited just above]. It is not nature which realizes freedom, but the concept of freedom which is realized in nature. The accomplishment of freedom and of the good Sovereign in the sensible world thus implies an original synthetic activity of man: History is this accomplishment, and thus it must not be confused with a simple development of nature. [44]

The final mediation between freedom of the will and "purposes" observable within nature is performed by judgment – that same faculty which gives us planetary man, species being in situ, and which only refers. It is in this place, in the third *Critique,* that we finally run across that long since familiar index of the human – "culture" – beyond, or in fact, lagging behind, the formality of the moral law. Notably, the treatment of culture in the *Critique of Judgment* does not reside in the aesthetic section, but in the section on teleology:

> Es bleibt also von allen seinen Zwecken in der Natur nur die formale, subjektive Bedingung, nämlich der Tauglichkeit: sich selbst überhaupt Zwecke zu setzen … (389).[45]
>
> It is a formal and subjective condition, namely mans aptitude in general for setting himself purposes … (319)
>
> *and*
>
> Die Hervorbringung der Tauglichkeit eines vernünftigen Wesens zu beliebigen Zwecken überhaupt (folglich in seiner Freiheit) ist die *Kultur.* (390).
>
> Producing in a rational being an aptitude for purposes generally (hence [in a way that leaves] that being free) is *culture.* (319)

In *Tauglichkeit*, a word also in military usage, one can hear echoes of "serviceability." "Aptitude" is in itself already useful, so that the autonomous (*beliebigen* – "free" or "arbitrary") relation to purposes that Pluhar glosses with "generally" (combining thereby *beliebig* and *überhaupt*) already includes a sort of undertow whereby this freedom of will will be reincorporated

44 Gilles Deleuze, *Kant's Critical Philosophy: The Doctrine of the Faculties*, trans. Hugh Tomlinson and Barbara Habberjam (Minneapolis: University of Minnesota Press, 1984), 74.

45 "Hence among all of his purposes in nature there remains only this [one], as that which nature can accomplish with a view to the final purpose outside of nature, and this [one] may therefore be regarded as nature's ultimate purpose: It is a formal and subjective condition, namely, man's aptitude in general for setting himself purposes." (319)

into the necessity of a general more general, an end more final or which, like Rousseau's individual will, will fall into step with the general. "Aptitude" also speaks to the sense of "suitability" in *Tauglichkeit* and to the semantic field that makes up one of its definitions: *eigen*. *Tauglichkeit* can also mean *geeignet sein* – but here again, the proper, even where it concerns freedom, is very close to being appropriated *angeeignet*. In the peculiarity of the genitival phrase in the original, the possibility arises that culture produces *by drawing forth or out of a rational being a particular form of serviceability*. Here again we encounter the tension between autonomous production and the task of reproducing forms. "Die Hervorbringung der Tauglichkeit eines vernünftigen Wesen zu beliebigen Zwecken überhaupt (folglich in seiner Freiheit) ist die *Kultur*." (The drawing forth of the servicability of a reasoning being for ends generally [in accordance with his freedom] is culture.)

It is not, of course, surprising that we soon thereafter read: "Aber nicht jede Kultur..." (*But not just any culture...*).[46] Whatever expectations concerning cultural specificity and diversity may have been raised by the thought of an investigation of aesthetic judgment (and equally disappointed) rush rather startlingly back to the fore in this distant entry to the Appendix of "Critique of Teleological Judgment," though here, too, the thought of the particular can only emerge via sweeping generality. Rather, through one more amplification of the subjective and formal, we arrive at a purely negative and formal concept of culture, a "constitution" (*Verfassung*) of human affairs *particularly* germane to the development of human culture in general.

> Die formale Bedingung, unter welcher die Natur diese ihre Endabsicht allein erreichen kann, ist diejenige Verfassung im Verhältnisse der Menschen untereinander, wo dem Abbruche der einander wechselseitig widerstreitenden Freiheit gesetzmässige Gewalt in einem Ganzen, welches bürgerliche Gesellschaft heißt, entgegengesetzt wird; denn nur in ihr kann die größte Entwickelung der Naturanlagen geschehen. (391)

> The formal condition under which nature can alone achieve this final aim is that constitution of human relations where the impairment to freedom which results from the mutually conflicting freedom [of the individuals] is countered by lawful authority within a whole called civil society. For only in this constitution of human relations can our natural predispositions develop maximally. (320)

Though in this passage *Verfassung* does not yet specifically imply the document of a "constitution," the resonance between the *Naturzweck* in the relation of its parts to Rousseau's elaboration of the general will is

46 "Aber nicht jede Kultur ist zu diesem letzten Zwecke der Natur hinlänglich" (390).

unmistakable. The "generative reflexivity" of diverse levels of formal definition have thus allowed the insinuation of a notion of *Bildungstrieb* to become an organizing or dominant metaphor within the appendix of the "Critique of Teleological Judgment." It is thus the species as a whole that must confront the greatest problem: the attainment of a civil society that can administer justice universally. Here again, a narrative or diachronic fusion with the structurally or synchronically exposed objects of teleological judgment performs its illusory, mediating function: the harmonization of divergent forms of lawfulness.

The formal definition of the activity of man includes the figure of the *Naturzweck* on two utterly distinct levels: first as the achievement of an organism-like structuring of human interactivity that assures a harmonious whole comprised of parts working in concert, but also as the end of ends that the *Naturzweck,* as an object of reflective judgment, prepares but *cannot be*. The *Naturzweck* thereby provides an index that cannot reach beyond the possibility it nonetheless constitutes.

* * *

If Kant's third *Critique* concerns itself with the particular – with the particular for which no general is given – how are we to conceive the possible nexus between judgments, organisms, or states of affair? To what extent are they particular? The heuristic use of analogy for purposes of observation starts to take on a *Bildungstrieb*-like activity whereby the example provided by Blumenbach, if only through virtue of generating new subsets of formal definition in the appendices, renders a model of civil "wholes" which are subject to becoming and which in their turn can define the human race in its becoming. We cannot determinately judge purposiveness in nature, but we can reflect it. This word takes on a double meaning because that faculty of judgment which gives itself an indeterminate law by which to subsume particulars relates structurally to the purposiveness it must assume in order to cognize natural purposes or organisms. Man, by being the natural purpose that can set itself purposes, embodies a purpose of nature by setting up the further formal manifestation of a will which a constitution protecting against the mutual contradiction of all individual wills would provide. In a formal and reflective way, the political goal of the Enlightenment is thus encapsulated in Kant's conceptualization of the research goals of its science. We might say that the nonwilling natural purpose provides a microcosmic duplicate, or offprint, of the culture of constitutions, so that in that sense the hexagon found in the sand, though at first comprising only potential evidence, could be argued to develop into a message or communiqué over the course of the appendix to the

Critique of Judgment.[47] It encodes a model of governance within the uncertain terrain of the developmental, the region of flux and untethered particularity. Between the grounded laws of the other two faculties' legislations, it offers a regulative idea or reflexive principle according to which a being could *guide its autonomy* and takes as its guide a very singular attribute of phenomena which felicitously mirrors judgment's own peculiar disposition. Here again the zone of reflective judgment presents a paradox whereby the formal definition of the supersensible freedom produces, via the reproductive faculty of the imagination, *something else*.

The Challenge of a General History

In a pair of earlier writings published in the *Berliner Monatsschrift* 6 years prior to the appearance of *Critique of Judgment*, "Idea for a Universal History with a Cosmopolitan Purpose" and "An Answer to the Question: 'What is Enlightenment?'" Kant had already conjectured on the possibility of the progress of reason in human history.[48] In these more popular writings we can find succinct statements of the question as to whether the "necessary freedom" of the moral law might be generalized for the species and in these essays too the figure of nature plays a pivotal role. If in *Critique of Judgment*, Kant proposes to at least *reflect* on the possibility of bridging the abyss between nature and freedom, here Kant tempts his audience with seeming reconciliations between the two, only to suggest through the style of the essays that recourse to appearances may remain insufficient in the face of the momentous question of the passage of freedom into human history. In particular, these popular essays conjure with the twin problems of: 1) observing *in general* and 2) *tracing* autonomy, each in its

47 The setter of purposes can will into being, in nature, that which is (the goal of) history. As Ernst Cassirer contends in his essay "Kant and Rousseau," both philosophers insist upon the self-constituting act of free wills in concert as the foundational political act. Though Kant may not share Rousseau's approach toward elaborating the general will, he follows Rousseau's basic assertion concerning the self-constitution of the political body. Cassirer cites Kant from the *Metaphysical Basis of the Theory of Law*: "'The act through which a people constitutes itself a state, or to speak more properly the *idea* of such an act, in terms of which alone its legitimacy can be conceived, is the original contract by which all (*omnes et singuli*) the people surrender their outward freedom in order to resume it at once as members of a common entity, that is, the people regarded as a state (universi).' Thus Kant achieved the same methodological transformation in the concept of the social contract as he had carried out in the interpretation of Rousseau's 'state of nature.' He transformed both form and 'experience' into an 'idea.'" (Cassirer, "Kant and Rousseau," 35).

48 Immanuel Kant, *Political Writings*, 41-60. German: Immanuel Kant, *Schriften zur Anthropologie* (Frankfurt am Main: Suhrkamp, 1996), 33-61. Henceforth, I will refer to these essays as "Idea for a Universal History" and "What is Enlightenment? "

own way posing a paradox for the possibility of a freedom not only rational, but also human.

As Foucault has noted, the essay contest which proposed the question, "What is Enlightenment?" bordered itself precariously on a present quickly becoming past, or to put it another way, a *becoming historical of the present.* Foucault writes,

> I find the question even more remarkable than the responses. For the "Enlightenment," at the end of this 18th century, was not new. It was not an invention, not a revolution, a party. It was something familiar and diffused which was in the process of happening and going away. The Prussian newspaper was basically asking: "What just happened to us? What is the event that is nothing other than what we have just said, thought and done – nothing other than ourselves, nothing other than this something that we were and that we still are?[49]

With his concise formulation, "If it is now asked whether we at present live in an *enlightened* age, the answer is: No, but we do live in an age of *enlightenment*," Kant's response to the essay question directly draws out a temporal dimension of the word "Aufklärung."[50] With the insistence on the distinction, Kant's text resists any understanding of enlightenment as a *concluded* process of self-reflection: only a procedural, ongoing self-reflection deserves the name. By refusing to consign enlightenment to the past Kant also, as Foucault points out further on in the same lecture, presents history itself as a challenge to philosophy.[51] And indeed, the question of progressive being-in-time forms the crux of the "What is Enlightenment?" essay as well as that of the "Idea for a Universal History." In the latter, Kant stops short of the historian's task of "narrating the appearances of a freedom of will in the history of human action" choosing instead to enumerate propositions that could be taken as the "Leitfaden" for

---

49 Opening passages of "For an Ethics of Discomfort" (*The Politics of Truth*, 135).

50 Kant, *Political Writings*, 58. Willi Goetschel argues that this formulation serves to distinguish enlightenment "not 'qualitatively' as *the* 'Enlightenment,' but at most 'quantitatively,' as an era of increasing enlightenment; instead of denoting a *perfectum* (of being already 'enlightened,' as the *Prolegomena* maintains [WW, 5:263; LWB, 130]), the word *enlightenment* [*Aufklärung*] thus shows itself to be a term of process, a progressive *substantivum*." Willi Goetschel, *Constituting Critique: Kant's Writing as Critical Praxis* (Durham: Duke University Press, 1994), 144-166.

51 "In short, in this text, it seems to me that one witnesses the appearance of the present as a philosophical event to which the philosopher who speaks about it belongs. … [A]nd I do not think that it is forcing things too much to say that for the first time, one sees philosophy problematize its own discursive actuality: an actuality that it questions as an event, as an event whose meaning, value, and philosophical singularity it has to express and in which it has to find both its own reason for being and the foundation for what it says." (*The Politics of Truth*, 86).

such a project in narration sometime in the future. The gesture of replacing *Erzählung* with *Satz* (proposition) thus writes itself, as theorem or proposition, out of time while still leaving the door open for a future work: It does not broach that historiography but speculatively founds the conditions of its possibility.

> Die Geschichte, welche sich mit der Erzählung dieser [Erscheinungen der Freiheit des Willens] beschäftigt, so tief auch deren Ursachen verborgen sein mögen, läßt dennoch von sich hoffen: daß, wenn sie das Spiel der Freiheit des menschlichen Willens *im großen betrachtet*, sie einen regelmäßigen Gang derselben entdecken könne ...[52]

> History is concerned with giving an account [*Erzählung*] of these phenomena, no matter how deeply concealed their causes may be, and it allows us to hope that, if it examines the free exercise of the human will *on a large scale*, it will be able to discover a regular progression among freely willed actions.[53]

In this passage from "Idea for a Universal History" the possibility for a formal generalization – human affairs regarded in general may expose a regular pattern – is presented by the same phrase "im großen" as it is in the subsequent essay "What is Enlightenment?" In the "Idea for a Universal History" essay, though, *observing in general* is presented as a direct possibility through reference to statistical representation, while in the second essay the adverbial phrase "im großen" ushers in a challenge to human understanding: human affairs, when regarded in general (*im großen*), show most everything to be paradoxical.[54] The difference between these two usages – the generality which reveals a pattern and the generality which reveals a paradox – could be glossed by distinguishing between biological and cultural reproduction: rates of birth, marriage and death versus the liberties assigned to teachers. In both cases, nonetheless, the curious problem presents itself that enlightenment – as potential attribute of the species and not only the rational agent – need also reproduce itself. How though would enlightenment reproduce? How would it retain the singularity of the rational agent while still reproducing that agent in history, across generations and from particular context to particular context, or even speaker to speaker?

In "Idea for a Universal History" *Sätze* (Propositions) 1-4 progressively fold the necessary (and purposive) development of the individual "creature" (*Geschöpfe*) into the species as presentable (or comprehensible)

52 Kant, *Werkausgabe*, vol. 11, 33.

53 Kant, *Political Writings*, 41.

54 See Rüdiger Campe, "Wahrscheinlich oder Scheinbar – mathematische Formel vs. philosophischer Diskurs (Quasi-Transzendental/Kant)" (*Spiel der Wahrscheinlichkeit*, 380-417) for a discussion of the role of the history of statistics in such a narration of scale.

as a moral whole [*ein moralisches Ganzes*].[55] This extends the operative model of the whole beyond the individual instance to a larger concert of wills.[56] The training of the purposes of reason in this account, however, necessarily exceed the span of one life and so, Kant argues, their eventuality thus cleaves to the species and not the individual: "so bedarf sie (Natur) einer vielleicht unabsehlichen Reihe von Zeugungen, deren eine der andern ihre Aufklärung überliefert" (*Zweiter Satz*) [it will require a long, perhaps incalculable series of generations, each passing on its enlightenment to the next].[57] From this point forward, the essay deploys the term "nature" as a metaphor for a process that instrumentalizes the *human being* in order to achieve her purposes in the *human species*. Such assertions run quite abruptly contrary to the account of the moral will, examined in the last chapter, which by definition *cannot suffer instrumentalization* (with the notable exception of marriage, itself one of the objects of statistical analysis with which the essay opens.).[58] In this proposal for a general or universal history, by contrast, we read:

> The highest task which nature has set for mankind must therefore be that of establishing a society in which *freedom under external laws* would be combined to the greatest possible extent with irresistible force [*Gewalt*], in other words of establishing a perfectly *just civil constitution* [*gerechte bürgerliche Verfassung*]. For only though the solution and fulfillment of this task can nature accomplish

55 Kant, *Political Writings*, 45. German: Kant, *Werkausgabe*, vol. 11, 38.

56 "Man kann die Geschichte der Menschengattung im großen als die Vollziehung eines verborgenen Planes der Natur ansehen, um eine innerlich- und, zu diesem Zwecke, auch äußerlich-vollkommene Staatsverfassung zu Stande zu bringen, als den einzigen Zustand, in welchem sie alle ihre Anlagen in der Menschheit völlig entwickeln kann. " Ibid., 45.

"The history of the human race as a whole can be regarded as the realisation of a hidden plan of nature to bring about an internally – and for this purpose also externally – perfect political constitution as the only possible state within which all natural capacities of mankind can be developed completely." Ibid., 50.

57 Ibid., 42-43. German: Ibid., 35-36.

58 In this respect, another sign of the "natural whole" as *Naturzweck* surreptitiously exerting its influence on the figuring of a moral whole will appear in §82 of the *Critique of Judgment*. There Kant writes, when strictly distinguishing between extrinsic and intrinsic purposiveness, "There is only one [case where] extrinsic purposiveness is connected with the intrinsic purposiveness of organization. This case is the organization of the two sexes as related to each other to propogate their species. Here, although we must not ask what is the end for which the being had to exist [as] so organized, [that being] still serves as a means extrinsically related to a purpose. For here, just as in the case of an individual, we can always go on to ask: Why did such a pair have to exist? The answer is: This pair is what first amounts to an *organizing* whole, even if not to an organized whole in a single body." (*Critique of Judgment*, 312-13) Here again a particular conception of embodiment announces trouble (or at least further complexity) for the analogy between the *Naturzweck* and the moral will, as well as for the desire to theorize a *species* enlightenment,and again in terms of reproduction. Put differently: *being for* another throws the ends of autonomy into paradox.

> its other intentions with our species. Man, who is otherwise so enamoured with unrestrained freedom, is forced [*zwingt*] to enter this state of restriction [*Zustand des Zwanges*] by necessity [*Not*] …[59]

The figure of instrumentalizing nature serves the function of producing a kind of Hobbesian spin on the fortunate fall: the selfish independence of the individual drives the individual, against his/her wishes, into a social state wherein pathological drives are gradually replaced with moral discernment.[60] This compulsion of nature can then unlock the natural *Anlagen* in the human faculties for acceding to freedom. In this account, the origins of *Kultur* take on an explicit formulation in paradox:

> All the culture and art which adorn mankind and the finest social order man creates are fruits of his unsociability. For it is compelled [*genötigt*] by its own nature to discipline itself, and thus, by enforced art [*abgedrungene Kunst*], to develop completely the germs [*Keime*] which nature implanted.[61]

The complex relation between the general and the particular in human judgment which will be investigated so thoroughly in the *Critique of Judgment* appears in these essays most frequently in organicist metaphors: seeds planted by nature will grow into enlightenment. The asociality prescribed by nature gradually turns into cultural progress through necessity, but in this process another paradox comes to light: the species becomes the subject of enlightenment, but even in this guise, "man" needs a master.

> Er bedarf also einen *Herrn*, der ihm den eigenen Willen breche, und ihn nötige, einem allgemein gültigen Willen, dabei jeder frei sein kann, zu gehorchen. Wo nimmt er aber diesen Herrn her? Nirgend anders als aus der Menschengattung. Aber dieser ist eben so wohl ein Tier, das einen Herrn nötig hat. Er mag es also anfangen, wie er will: so ist nicht abzusehen, wie er sich ein Oberhaupt der öffentlichen Gerechtigkeit verschaffen könne, das selbst gerecht sei ...

> He thus requires a *master* to break his self-will and force him to obey a universally valid will under which everyone can be free. But where is he to find such a master? Nowhere else but in the human species.[62] But this master will also be an animal who needs a master. Thus while man may try as he will, it is hard to see how he can obtain for public justice a supreme authority which would itself be just …[63]

---

59 Kant, *Political Writings*, 45-46. German: Kant, *Werkausgabe*, vol. 11, 39.

60 See Adorno on the multiple meanings of "nature" in Kant and their bearing on his moral philosophy. Theodor Adorno, *Problems of Moral Philosophy*, trans. Rodney Livingstone (Stanford: Stanford University Press, 2001), 89-95.

61 Kant, *Political Writings*, 46. German: Kant, *Werkausgabe*, vol. 11, 40.

62 Kant, *Political Writings*, 46.

63 Kant, *Political Writings*, 46.

Beyond the almost homonymic repetition of "Herrn her" which threatens to render the question absurd, Kant also point to the doubling of "man" that the history of freedom *as general history* will require. There is as yet no "example" of such a general history as he avers in the Eighth Proposition – but in this passage Kant condenses certain paradoxes of the will central to its possibility. The agent of history, *der Mensch*, "needs a master to break his own will for him": the temporary suspension of the very freedom that provides the only possibility for the eventuality of enlightenment. Thanks to the syntactical arrangement of the sentence particular to the German language the sentence could also read: "such that each can be free ... to obey" (*jeder frei sein kann zu gehorchen*). We cannot necessarily admit of this reading – as Kant emphasized in his essay in response to the question: "not even Caesar is above the grammarians" – and yet the antithesis nonetheless inheres in a possible vocalization of the sentence. Further, the paradox extends into the institutions of governance: Though the species becomes lord, no single member of it stands outside the need to be mastered, and the irresistible force of the general will thus reveals itself not only in terms of the principle of contradiction but also as material force (*Gewalt*).

Here, the reader can intimate the blend of theoretical and ethical questions that will come to comprise the heuristic use of reflective judgment in *Critique of Judgment.* In the transition from the Sixth to the Seventh Proposition (a gap interestingly undergirded by a footnote concerning the possible comparison of human beings to the inhabitants of other planets), the problem of the endurance of a Hobbesian state of nature replicates itself in the dilemma presented by the aggression *between* states: what will happen if one general will encounters another? (And so on and so on…) Here, through brief reference to Epicurus, the essay suggests that the question as to whether political history be construed as a product of accident, a movement of progress or potential degeneration can be summed up (*hinausläuft*) in the question: "Whether it is rational to assume that the order of nature is *purposive* in its parts but *purposeless* as a whole." Interestingly, the figure of nature as the catalyst for man's *becoming historical* or becoming the agent of history runs into the problem of competing totalities. The conception of a final totality figurally counteracts the problem of infinite regress, but only limited models of purpose can guide reflection without recurring to a teleology that becomes theology. Under what circumstances and at what cost can we apply purposiveness to nature as a whole and thus impute a purpose to history? This question renders in condensed form a question that will be taken on in a much expanded form in the closing sections of *Critique of Judgment.*

While "Idea for a Universal History" demures before writing a narrative of universal history (claiming that it is waiting for "nature" to "bring forth" the man capable of writing it), Kant's essay on enlightenment addresses its public directly, not querying the possibility of progress, but on the contrary, asking: in what cases is it legitimate to *defer* the progress (*Fortschreiten*: the substantivation of the German verb which vividly includes the image of "stepping out") of enlightenment? With this negative articulation of the question, Kant moves between the scientific and juridical meanings of the word law, answering empathically that to prevent the progressive development of man's *Naturanlagen* would be a crime against humanity. The two essays, when taken together and compared, reflect a branching in Kant's lines of inquiry: "Idea for a Universal History," on the one hand, proposes history as an effect of nature, of the pressure of instincts and their metamorphosis; "What is Enlightenment?" on the other, contemplates history as a product of human legislation and argument. The exit constituted by a stepping forth in the essay "What is Enlightenment?" shifts the terms of opposition from that between *Geschöpf* and *Gattung*, the operative categories of the "Idea for a Universal History" essay, to those of *ein einzelner Mensch* and *ein Publikum*. In the "What is Enlightenment?" essay the transition into the collective singular takes place when the plural "sie," which refers to the non-autonomous, unenlightened group of the opening paragraphs, is subsumed by the organizing principle of *a public*: "Daß aber ein Publikum sich selbst aufkläre, ist eher möglich; ja es ist, wenn man ihm nur Freiheit läßt, beinahe unausbleiblich." (*That a public would enlighten itself is more probable. Indeed, when left to freedom, it is almost inevitable.*)[64] In this permutation of the dichotomy between general and particular, the problem of reproduction moves from the sphere of species reprodutcion (statistics of birth, marriage and death rates: *Geschöpf: Gattung*) to that of the function of pedagogy (various institutions of church and state described in terms of their mechanicity). These institutions, though their necessity is avowed, interestingly lose their place as *telos* of human history in the transaction. In "What is Enlightenment?" the inevitability of what could be termed the "reproduction of the social sphere" – a progeneration (*Zeugung*) bent on tradition or inheritance (*Überlieferung*) of cultural forms – is both acknowledged and limited: set within its proper sphere.

The role of the figure of reproduction thus becomes quite complex, since on the one hand the docile student of doctrine becomes a kind of

64 Kant, *Werkausgabe*, vol. 11, 54. English: Reese translation. In this instance, the Nisbet translation unfortunately takes the emphasis off the word "public": "There is more chance of an entire public enlightening itself. This is indeed almost inevitable, if only the public concerned is left in freedom." (*Political Writings*, 55)

Hausvieh, repeating cant, while on the other, the species and its government require this. A doubling of temporal lines ensues in that precepts and rules reproduce themselves almost automatically across the populace while gradually individual members of a public step forth beyond such guidelines. Kant writes that they move clear of the *Gängelwagen* of prescription and prejudice, a term also used in the *First Critique* when describing the practice of judgment and the utility of example. Though the double attribution of the individual as both passive member (*passives Glied*) and self-enlightening agent points to what many have regarded as the somewhat sorry circumscription of the field of action Kant secures for enlightenment, the distinction also surprisingly reverses the terms of "freedom of conscience" insisting instead on public address.[65]

> So fern sich aber dieser Teil der Maschine zugleich als Glied eines ganzen gemeinen Wesens, ja sogar der Weltbürgergesellschaft ansieht, mithin in der Qualität eines Gelehrten, der sich an ein Publikum im eigentlichen Verstande durch Schriften wendet: Kann er allerdings räsonnieren, ohne daß dadurch die Geschäfte leiden, zu denen er zum Teile als passives Glied angesetzt ist.[66]

> But in so far as this or that individual who acts as part of the machine also considers himself as a member of a complete commonwealth or even of cosmopolitan society, and thence as a man of learning who may through his writings address a public in the truest sense of the word, he may indeed argue without harming the affairs in which he is employed for some of the time in a passive capacity.[67]

In Kant's German the distinction between these two capacities is not phrased "passive part of the time" but rather "part, in part." To paraphrase: *Er ist Teil zum Teile*. In part part of the machine but simultaneously member of a whole, collective entity as (passive) member (*zugleich als [passives] Glied*). This double individual is "employed" (also applied, joined, set or started). The simultaneity of these two separate distinctions casts the earthly institutions which circumscribe conduct as mere extensions of the domestic sphere.

> Thus the use which someone employed as a teacher makes of his reason in the presence of his congregation is purely *private*, since a congregation, however large it is, is never any more than a domestic [*häusliche*] gathering. In

65 Foucault, *The Politics of Truth*, 108. See Willi Goetschel's compelling account of the role of this publication and others both in public response to Kant's sovereign, Frederick II, and within his larger conception of reason. (*Constituting Critique*, 145-153)

66 Kant, *Werkausgabe*, vol. 11, 56.

67 Kant, *Political Writings*, 56.

> view of this, he is not and cannot be free as a priest, since he is acting on a commission imposed from outside [*einen fremden Auftrag richtet*].[68]

The maintenance of religious and civil institutions takes on a machinic aspect and a feminization much akin to that of Dr. Frankenstein when building his daemon's female other. The authority of the clergy amounts to mere reproduction. Further, the somewhat counterintuitive phrasing of the passage builds a paradox: as member of the inner, private group he is burdened with a task imposed from without, a foreign duty or duty not inherent in his will. With the introduction of the term *Volk*, however, another collective singular enters the discussion and the dichotomy between the individual and a public is trined. In this case, *ein Volk* (and not a species) forms the figure of an entity alienated from its agency, not yet autonomous, but also invoked in an amplification of the categorical imperative to offer the fiction of a test case. The Volk becomes the protagonist of a fiction whereby a collective exercise of the categorical imperative could provide a *Probierstein* of justice.

> To test whether any particular measure can be agreed upon as a law for a people, we need only ask whether a people could well impose such a law upon itself.[69]

> Der Probierstein alles dessen, was über ein Volk als Gesetz beschlossen werden kann, liegt in der Frage: ob ein Volk sich selbst wohl ein solches Gesetz auferlegen könnte?[70]

Here, much in constrast to the essay "Idea for a Universal History," which addresses itself explicitly to the philosophy of history, we discover that progressive enlightenment (not identical presumably to the arrival of freedom but conducive thereof) constitutes a point of origin. The furtherance of critical knowledge, "eine ursrpüngliche Bestimmung" in which human nature consists (and not just as seed or *Anlage* to be awakened through repression), becomes the self-generating origin of enlightenment. Where in the "Idea for a Universal History" essay Kant left a gap between "proposition" and "narration," the enlightenment essay construes that gap as a kind of temporal disjunction within the agent. Though on the one hand, the administers of culture hum along like parts of a machine, on the other, they must be able to act in the speculative sphere of a self-imposed legislation: the idea of keeping the guardians of the people as immature as the people itself "ist eine Ungereimtheit, die auf Verewigung der Ungereimtheiten hinausläuft." The figure of an absurdity running off into infin-

68 Kant, *Political Writings,* 57.

69 Kant, *Political Writings*, 57.

70 Kant, *Werkausgabe*, vol. 11, 58.

ity here caps the possibility of a completely enclosed reproducibility of knowledge.

Together with the phrase "im großen," we see here another operative figure of speech that spans the two essays. The running of questions or phrases either into infinity or into imponderable questions build the structural field of limiting regresses within which Kant composes his inquiry. Posed across from one another *in general*, as pattern and paradox, and *hinauslaufen*, as a turn of phrase which conjures something like a vanishing point, both suggest the kind of chiasmus which Kant's discourse builds but doesn't always state. That man needs a master and can only find that master in one who himself needs a master leads us to the possibility that a collective could be figured as a whole formed by a concert of self-determining wills. The problem reduplicates itself, however, when one such whole confronts another and ever burgeoning spheres of aggressive competition ensue "amounting" or "running up" to the question of a broader purpose in history. General history thus broaches the near impossible hope of proposing an encompassing whole which does not succumb to replication and spiraling conflict. Across from this, delimiting the reasoning power of the "guardians of the people" itself amounts to the eternaliztion of absurdities. Here Kant plays on the root "Mund" in the two words: if the *Vormünder des Volkes* should themselves be *unmündig* then we have arrived at an absurdity, or insist upon the identity of a contradiction. The enlightenment essay which *answers* and doesn't just propose, strongly privileges speech in the figure of the mouth. Still, the touch stone of a law's justice remains in the *question* as to whether a people *could* impose such a law on itself, thus transposing the people into a reflexive figure not yet come into being but voiced through a surrogate disembodied questioner.

* * *

In an illuminating reading of Kant's essay on universal history Rüdiger Campe suggests that with his reference to statistics Kant plays on the double meaning of the word *Spiel* (to mean both theatrical production and game of chance) partly by way of the double meaning of *im großen* in this one text.[71] Moreover, Campe points out that these two meanings of *Spiel*

71 Man findet hier zwei verschiedene Konstellationen aus Regellosigkeit und Regel: Die Statistik sieht im Spiel, das *im großen* abläuft, von vornherein sich wiederholende Handlungen, kulturelle Repertoires (Sterben, Heiraten, Gebären). Von Seiten der praktischen Kritik erinnert Kant hier an die Singularität der jeweils einzelnen moralischen Handlung, die in den abzählbaren Handlungsrepertoires unverrechenbar verborgen liegt. (2) Das Spiel *im großen*, das auf der Bühne spielt, meint dagegen gerade einzelne Handlungen. Freilich nicht

remain consonant for a tradition running as far as Leibniz or Pascal, in that the hidden plan of providence – what one would see if provided a glimpse behind the curtains – reintroduces the possibility of a regulation of chaos through divine justice, allowing that the world's stage as well as that of the game of chance house the same form of contingency. Kant's critical philosophy, however, interupts this continuum, dividing the two contingent forms and introducing a lack into discursive philosophy which finds need of the *figure* of statistical representation as its supplement.

Campe's reading makes powerful arguments as to the simultaneously presupposed and disavowed role of statistical probability for Kant's critical philosophy: though not accepted as an evidential form of knowledge, statistics inform Kant's critique, as the *image* of evidence without which they cannot function.[72] For Campe's reading, the return of statistical probability in the third *Critique* and short essay "Idea for a Universal History" thus becomes instructive given the prior exclusion of statistics from the realms of both pure (theoretical) and practical reason. By becoming the operatively excluded term, statistical findings present to *Critique of Judgment* the *image* of that which cannot actually be apprehended. The suggestion, however, that "Idea for a Universal History" relies on this, perhaps disavowed, gesture toward the statistically presentable overlooks the possibility that Kant's refusal to narrate a universal history might constitute an affirmation of sorts. By refusing the perfect mapping of political being onto species being – leaving the gap open – Kant can describe enlightenment man as both continuous with and distinct from anthropological man. Deferring narration, therefore, offers an innovation of form akin to the architectonics of the critical philosophy itself. Questions housed at the limits delineated by antinomy, infinite regress and the vanishing point of reason's reflexivity preserve the space for a questioning of causation which leaves the paradoxes presented by competing forms of universality intact.

---

in ihrem moralischen Freiheitscharakter sind sie hier betrachtet, sondern als Aktionen, aus denen Geschichten und Geschichte bestehen. Eine Planhaftigkeit, die man unterstellen könnte, müßte in diesem Fall aus dem Zusammenhang hergenommen werden, den die Geschichte und ihre Erzählung liefert. Eine allgemeine und philosophische Geschichte gibt es nur, wenn man beide Konstellationen wie ein einziges Feld von Ereignissen behandelt. Genau das tut Kants *Idee einer allgemeinen Geschichte*. (*Wahrscheinlichkeit*, 406)

72 Such a reading offers an extension of the understanding, proferred by Kant himself, that the work of *Critique of Judgment* is to mediate between the abyss dividing the the first two critiques, that between theoretical and practical philosophy, or freedom and nature. Campe notes that the two most remarkable references to statistical analysis in Kant's oeuvre are found in passages treating of judgment, one with respect to aesthetics and the other with respect to philosophy of history. (*Wahrscheinlichkeit*, 389)

The Encyclopeadic and the Propadeutic

Already in *Critique of Pure Reason*, it is the impossibility of drawing the law of natural causality to the level of the universal that offers the first indication of an alternate form of causality in freedom. Since the law of nature requires that "nothing can happen without a sufficient *a priori* determined cause," there cannot be "any real beginning of things," because each first cause would require an antecedent cause.[73] Thus to assume natural law as universal leads to infinite regress and contradiction. As Kant writes:

> Hence the proposition, in its unlimited universality (*unbeschränkten Allgemeinheit*), whereby any causality is possible only according to natural laws contradicts itself; and hence this causality cannot be assumed as being the only one. (474)[74]

Unexpectedly, the thesis (asserting a causality beyond that of the laws of nature) safeguards the grounds of freedom, for the exclusive application of natural law founders on self-contradiction, while its opposite only fails to present itself to experience.[75] As Adorno notes in his lectures on moral philosophy, the self-contradiction entailed by the universalization of natural law in the Thesis of the "Third Conflict of Transcendental Ideas" reveals both how early in Kant's work the problem of practical philosophy announces itself, but also how "Kant ... establishes transcendental freedom on the basis of the causality of nature." Once again, the argument here moves through an exposition of limits and an impasse leads to an unexpected expansion. We might say that through the contradiction generated by the extension of the natural law of causality to the universal, transcendental freedom finds its surprising grounds. The bind of the antinomy extends the concept of causality to include "causality born of freedom" (*Kausalität aus Freiheit*) with the result that freedom, in its necessity, remains ineluctably connected, for its demonstration, to the limiting case of the theoretical sphere, or causality in nature.[76]

---

73 Kant, *Critique of Pure Reason*, 484.

74 Immanuel Kant, *Critique of Pure Reason*, trans. Werner S. Pluhar (Indianapolis: Hackett, 1996), 474. German: Immanuel Kant, *Kritik der reinen Vernunft* (Leipzig: Verlag von Feliz Meiner, 1930), 463.

75 Henry Allison, *Kant's Theory of Freedom* (New York: Cambridge University Press, 1990), 20.

76 Here Kant's readers diverge markedly, and it is true that by following Adorno, I follow a particularly partisan, though astonishingly attentive and creative reader. While Kant resolves the antinomy by allowing that a cause other to natural laws would be intelligible rather than empirical, Adorno shows little patience with this outcome. On one of the few occasions on which one of the authors of *Dialectic of Enlightenment* makes an appearance, Adorno remarks as to this "resolution": "What I am concerned about is that you should understand from the outset that the contradiction we are confronted with is not, as Kant

Kant's readers take up markedly different positions on both the status and the future (within later works) of the third antinomy.[77] Adorno attributes its legacy to the "peculiar Janus-face of Kantian philosophy":

> You can see, on the one hand, how he is driven by his own analysis to the realization that giving any such absolute status to the primal thing – whether it be the category of causality or that of the freedom that necessarily precedes it – leads inexorably to contradictions that prove to be insoluble. On the other hand, he nevertheless refuses to relinquish the idea of something absolute and primary. This leads him – and this is why this issue is so important for practical philosophy – by a *coup de main* to establish freedom as a law *sui generis* that then stands absolutely at the beginning, conferring a sort of primacy on practical reason.[78]

The antithesis and the possibility of the sudden and unprepared "origin of a cause" in freedom bears importantly upon the various articulations of enlightenment we have been considering in the essays Kant offered to the wider reading public in the 1780's. The strange doubling of an enlightening subject between reproducer of doctrine and author of public discourse, along with Kant's refusal to narrate a history of freedom, point to temporal incongruities and paradoxes associated with the causality of freedom in his account.

The early imbrication of freedom, nature and necessity in Kant's thinking of causality could be said to generate the gap or abyss within which his philosophy moves. Much of the work undertaken in the wake of his ethics engages just this: repeated attempts to articulate the intelligible but supersensual concept of freedom with respect to time and in history. In these reworkings and rethinkings crucial legacies of what we mean by "culture" are to be divined, though shot through with the persistent concept of nature, and often in our own forgetting of the paradoxes of origin in which they are suspended.

As we have seen, the necessity for human judgment to adjudicate in terms of purposes serves to generate a purely formal definition of culture

---

would have us believe in the 'Solution,' a contradiction that results from our inadequate use of causality, but is rather, a contradiction that arises because things in the world by their own meaning necessarily become caught up in this contradiction." Adorno finds Kant, in this instance, to come close to the later positivists who advise: "Behave from the outset like bureaucrats who refuse to lift a finger to do any work that is outside their department …," (*Problems of Moral Philosophy*, 45-46).

77 For a recent reading of note that traces the concept of freedom through the series of Kant's philosophy see Michelle Kosch, *Freedom and Reason in Kant, Schelling, and Kierkegaard* (Oxford: Clarendon Press, 2006). Of particular importance for my discussion is Chapter 4 in Eckart Förster's *Kant's Final Synthesis*, though Förster's argument takes its point of departure from "the idea of a moral world." Eckart Förster, *Kant's Final Synthesis*, 118-26.

78 Adorno, *Problems of Moral Philosophy*, 47.

as the structural figure for a history of freedom. In this respect, *Critique of Judgment* does present a powerful vision of cultural making – despite its lack of interest in the history of art – but this making doesn't so much produce a work as an aptitude (*Tauglichkeit*), usefulness or suitability. Interestingly, the word *Tauglichkeit* emerges at two pivotal points of Kant's exposition of teleological judgment: first, with respect to the formal purposiveness exhibited by geometrical figures and then again in the definition of culture we have considered. Kant eschews the value of the usefulness of geometrical figures, pointing to the ancient philosophical tradition which studied geometry on its own merits, not predicting that it would have such a wide range of future utility. Of the ancient geometers he writes,

> It is a true joy to see how eagerly the ancient geometers investigated these properties of such lines (in this case, conic sections), not letting themselves be disconcerted if asked by narrow minds of what use such knowledge might be. Thus they investigated the properties of the parabola without knowing the law of terrestrial gravitation, which would have allowed them to apply the parabola to the trajectory of heavy bodies ... While these geometers were thus unwittingly working for posterity, they took delight in a purposiveness which, though it belonged to the nature [*Wesen*] of things, could still be exhibited completely a priori in its necessity. ... For there is a necessity in what is purposive and of such a character [that it seems] as if it had intentionally been so arranged for our use, while yet it also seems to belong to the original nature [*Wesen*] of things, without any concern as to [how] we might use it; and this necessity is the basis for our great admiration of nature [*Natur*], not so much nature outside us as nature in our own reason. (240-241, 308-309)

Thus, even the geometrical figure, which *can become* serviceable for theoretical reason maintains its own purposeless purposiveness and must be retained on the side of the *a priori*. Further, Kant maintains that when "I draw a figure *in accordance with a concept,* I *introduce* the *purposiveness into* the figure, i.e., into my own way of presenting something that is given to me from outside, whatever it may be in itself, rather than this something's instructing me empirically about that purposiveness." (242, 311). The imputation of purposiveness, together with the indication of alternate forms of understanding implicit in it, make it crucial for the third *Critique* to hold to the "Antinomy of Judgment" and refuse to assume a *real* purposiveness in material bodies. If our construction of nature is to reflect adequately the unique formation of our judgment, the purposive structure must remain a product of the imagination and only tentatively impute the possibility of such an organizing structure to natural beings. We must *introduce* purposiveness into the world while suspending the thought of its future applicability in natural science. Interestingly, the example Kant offers of a "real purposiveness" is a garden.

> This is different from cases where I find order and regularity in an aggregate, enclosed within certain boundaries, of *things* outside me: e.g. in a garden, order and regularity among trees, flower beds, walks, etc. For in these cases I cannot hope to infer a priori this order and regularity from the way I have bounded a space in accordance with this or that rule. (242, 310)

To assume real purposiveness in the *Naturzweck*, and thus to determine it, would be to construe nature as a garden and teleology, as Kant notes, when taken to its furthest application, becomes theology. Nonetheless, the hexagon in the sand – the primary figure of Kant's speculative fiction concerning the problem posed by the pattern and regularity of nature for our understanding offers a spur of sorts to continue seeking formative principles within the aggregate of natural laws, even when this leads us beyond the immediate capacities of our own understanding.

The virtualization of concept-formation of which the reflective judgment is capable generates models for ethicotheology but is operating in an exiled application of theoretical reason and absolutely limited in its sphere of determining objects. One could say that just as aesthetic judgment entails *zwecklose Zweckmäßigkeit*, teleological judgment brought in its train "particularity-less particularity." It could conceptualize a coming of freedom into nature, but not assure or anchor it beyond a formal universality. As we have also observed, this formal universality can be brought to generate a certain form of historical content with respect to a culture of constitutions, a form of governance predicated on the "idea" Kant makes of Rousseau's general will. This is the move made in "Idea for a Universal History." In that essay, though, the formality of the purposive totality is alloyed with the supplement of a figure of nature which instrumentalizes the individual human agent beyond it's own representations (*Vorstellungen*).

With the autonomously productive generation of purposive totalities in the critique of teleological judgment, Kant avoids predicating nature along the lines taken in "Idea for a Universal History" (or in *Religion within the Boundaries of Mere Reason*, for that matter). Though he does briefly reiterate the arguments of "Idea for a Universal History" in §83 of the Appendix to "Critique of Teleological Judgment," the harmonization of the formal structures struck up between the definition of a *Naturzweck* and governance via *Verfassung* constitutes by far the more evocative and predominant strain in the work. Further, the heuristic investigation of a *possible* theory of biological forms – which though it may tempt the divide between theoretical and practical does not transgress it – clearly throws its weight behind the future of an empirical, natural science in opposition to the kind of speculation that will come to characterize the ensuing idealist tradition.

One could nonetheless wonder, whether Kant were not also testing out possible modes of commensuration between two forms of reason, practical and theoretical, by proposing these virtual experiments with the concept of the purposive. A point made in Adorno's lectures on moral philsophy contributes here to an interpretation of the particular form of relation between practical and theoretical reason attributable to the critique of teleological judgment:

> And I believe that if you want to go back to the origins of what Kant actually meant by freedom, if you want to obtain a precise picture of the model that underlies his concept of freedom, a concept which in general we use in a fairly casual, imprecise manner, then it will turn out to be simply this remarkable faculty that enables us to organize in our imagination the various components of the natural world or of existing reality, and to rearrange them in different ways from those in which we found them initially and in which they exist in reality. This fact, this readily observable fact, that in its origins and its content mind points back to nature, but at the same time is not reducible to it, is, I believe, what Kant probably means by this entire doctrine of freedom in the midst of nature.[79]

On the one hand, Adorno goes on to argue that such a position is not tenable within the either-or logic with which Kant operates and insists that only a dialectical logic could accommodate such an understanding of freedom. On the other, and at various junctures of his lectures, Adorno points to an alternate mode for confronting contradiction in Kant's philosophy. He sees moments of breaking off in Kant's philosophy as evidence of an ongoing process of revision and self-correction.[80] While Kant's contemporaries and successors were often to grow impatient with these points of "rupture" within his architectonic, it is quite likely that it is precisely this practice of philosophizing that allows it to possess what Adorno aptly designates as "a consciousness of non-identity" such that reason sets the limit upon itself whereby it cannot construe itself as the origin of everything that exists.[81]

> Paradoxically, then, even though Kant criticized heteronomy so fiercely, everything that is non-ego, and is thereby heteronomous, is more revered in a certain sense and is allowed to assert itself more powerfully than in the idealist philosophies. The latter do indeed concede a greater recognition of the

---

79 Adorno, *Problems of Moral Philosophy*, 103.

80 Ibid., 55, 59 and 95.

81 Ibid., 96.

non-ego than does Kant, but since they absorb it into the ego, in effect they dissolve it there and hence strive to vindicate and legitimate it as rational.[82]

To insist too empatically on the generative possibilities revealed in teleological judgment by the observation – provided by natural beauty – of the imagination operating autonomously (according to rules its assigns to itself) and generating generalities where none so far exist would risk once again closing the gap or abyss. Indeed it is likely that Kant turns to the notion of radical evil in his next work, *Religion innerhalb der Grenzen der bloßen Vernunft*, not only because *Critique of Judgment* still leaves adherence to moral duty largely without incentive and assurance, but also because the conjectures based on the *Naturzweck*, as Förster argues, still do not sufficiently concern the "realization of a moral world."[83] Further, in this reader's view, they threaten to harmonize the moral will too fully with the organic model, "the appearance of a will" in virtual forms of immanent teleology. (Thus the ambiguity and exegetical challenge of Kant's reference to the human will as a "natural cause" in section 2 of the second introduction.) It is possible that the desire for a transition through the abyss does not also allow a retroactive erasure thereof, especially not where one is engaged with the paradoxes of identity in time, temporal becoming.[84] Aesthetic judgment suspended the subjective universality of

---

82 Ibid.

83 Förster, *Kant's Final Synthesis*, 131. See also 130-135.

84 In *Religion within the Boundaries of Mere Reason*, Kant proposes a distinction between "intelligible action," construed as an action cognizable by reason alone, and "sensible action," construed as an action given in time. Immanuel Kant, *Werkeausgabe*, vol. 8, 689. English: Immanuel Kant, *Religion within the Boundaries of Mere Reason*, ed. and trans. Allen Wood and George di Giovani (New York: Cambridge University Press, 1998), 55. Where *Critique of Judgment* could be argued to erect a structure of contradictions from within which the reader must imagine the paradoxical attainment of freedom in nature, *Religion* argues rationally for something of a mystery in the distinction between intelligible and sensible acts. Kant's account of an origin of religion within morality once again resolves upon certain contradictions that arise in his moral thought, for "we cannot … inquire into the origin in time of this deed but must inquire only into its origin in reason. " (63) German: 691. Interestingly, the scene of narrating origin stories provides this argument with an instance of a rational reflection that must assent to an origin which cannot be located determinately in historical time – other than *now*, ("it still is his duty, now") – and which itself can offer a detemporalized account of an origin, in this case of religion from morality and not the contrary. [See Part 1, Section 4] (Ibid.) Even in his own improvisatory contribution to the genre of 18th century philosophical fictions, or speculative origin stories, "Mutmaßlicher Anfang der Menschengeschichte," (*Conjectures on the Beginning of Human History*) Kant will portray not only his own such fiction but in a concluding remark will point to his own reader as the speculator who will, in a reasoned act, actually choose this story as reason's history and thus affirm the account through a representation of reason. In this sense, Kant too, along with Shelley and Kleist either scripts the story of origin in the historical present – or outside of time altogether. In both *Critique of Judgment* and *Religion within the Boundaries of*

taste between the two imperatives "you must try it out" and "you must make a claim on universal assent" in keeping with the peculiarly productive sphere of a regulative principle (akin to the *a priori* knowledge of the supersensible freedom in the moral philosophy).[85] Such a simultaneously *a priori* and temporally conditioned tie to empirical testing presented a form of necessity that enables Kant's *Critique of Judgment* to reach toward the paradox of a "general history" of "culture" understood as a purely formal affair. As was the case in the essay "An Idea for a Universal History," here too, Kant prefers a structure of principles to narration. Thus the two central contradictions of the third *Critique*:

> Aber die Möglichkeit einer lebenden Materie (deren Begriff einen Widerspruch enthält, weil Leblosigkeit, inertia, den wesentlichen Charakter derselben ausmacht) läßt sich nicht einmal denken...
>
> And yet we cannot even think of living matter as possible. (The [very] concept of it involves a contradiction, since the essential character of matter is lifelessness, [in Latin] *inertia.*)
>
> *and*
>
> Allein daß die Einbildungskraft frei und doch von selbst gesetzmäßig sei, d.i. daß sie eine Autonomie bei sich führe, ist ein Widerspruch. Der Verstand allein gibt das Gesetz. (160)
>
> And yet, to say that the *imagination* is *free* and yet *lawful of itself*, i.e., that it carries autonomy with it, is a contradiction. The understanding alone gives the law. (91)

stand across from one another, divided by the line between aesthetic and teleological judgment. In the field produced by their mutual reflection, they generate a space within which matter becomes a virtual index and feeling makes a demand upon the empirical world. Kant's carefully wrought critique thus produces a field of antinomies (aporias) that must be crossed through by the reader, and a harmonizing of forms of lawful-

---

Mere Reason freedom necessitates this paradoxical double identity of an act. In the latter, I fear that the pith of action is cast utterly out of the world, whereas in the former the paradox leads to the outcome that critique cannot stand outside of history but must actively constitute it. Kant, *Political Writings*, 221-234.

85 In the second introduction to the *Critique of Judgment*, Kant makes the following statement about the concept of freedom: "The very concept of freedom carries with it, as far as nature is concerned, only a negative principle (namely, of mere opposition), but gives rise to expansive principles for the determination of the will, which are therefore called practical ...". (9-10). "Da nun die ersteren ein *theoretisches* Erkenntnis nach Prinzipien a priori möglich machen [Naturbegriffe], der zweite [Der Freiheitsbegriff] aber in Ansehung derselben nur ein negatives Prinzip (der bloßen Entgegensetzung) schon in seinem Begriffe bei sich führt, dagegen für die Willensbestimmung erweiternde Grundsätze, welche darum praktisch heißen, errichtet..." (78).

ness that must be *actively imagined.* Similarly, the pivotal section on the peculiar limitation of human understanding as predicated upon the distinction between actual and possible enters the critique in Section §76 with nothing but the title "Comment." The exposition of this important point, Kant asserts, must wait for full explanation and for the moment can only be stated "episodish" or digressively. The many levels of mirroring which *Critique of Judgment* thus structures, between its parts, between judgment and the possibility of experience it constitutes, between the particular instance and the general rule, between individuals and species, beween agents and collectivities, challenge its interpreter to the kind of reflective-making its critique discloses. The reader's activity in this is both paramount, though to some extent already foreclosed, by the stasis of the structures of contradictions which have been put into place. The distinction between possible and actual doesn't only characterize human understanding, it also opens the space for freedom, though the elaboration of that space itself becomes a kind of vanishing act.

In the first, unpublished introduction to *Critique of Judgment*, Kant delineates a distinction between two forms of introduction, the propadeautic and the encylcopeadic. Notably, the propadeutic, which would ordinarily precede an individual work, would not make any claim on presenting (or introducing) a comprehensive systematicity. The encyclopeadic, in contrast, could only follow a concluded and total systematization, explaining how the work to come fits in with the total system. Despite his consistent commitment to the maintenance of clear distinctions, however, Kant immediately proposes to violate this one.

> Now the power whose own principle we are here trying to discover and discuss – the power of judgment – is of a very special kind. ... Therefore, as I determine the principles of such a power – one that is fit not for a doctrine but merely for a critique – I may be permitted to depart from the order that is indeed necessary elsewhere, and to begin [rather than conclude] with a brief encyclopaedic introduction of judgment ... In this way I shall combine the propaedeutic introduction with the encylopeadic one. (432)

In keeping with the peculiar autonomy of reflective judgment explored in *Critique of Judgment*, the finish must proceed the start and embarkation can only be undertaken through the reflection of already conceived ends. Further, this heterogeneity of the introduction points to the temporal paradoxes necessary for Kantian critique to take organic form, history or culture as its object.

Caught in the hinge of the temporal paradoxes of Kant's presentation of aesthetic judgment and the possibility of a general history, or a history of freedom, remains the intransigent question of reproduction. Much as

Dr. Frankenstein's monster intruded on the pure mirroring between general and individual wills as an utterly contingent, embodied *fact* of politics, the contradictory autonomy of the imagination and of observed living matter subtends *Critique of Judgment.* The reproductive spheres of imagination and species-life prove an utterly indispensable – even if often disavowed – companion to the *a priori* which heralds from the realms of the contingent. This possibility is even more pronounced in the first introduction wherein speciation provides the principle of judgment that causes form itself to become raw substrate. In disclosing the most exemplary example, the double being of species life signals the work of the contingent in the precincts of the necessary and cannot be overlooked.

As in the case of the essay "What is Enlightenment?" enlightenment must remain disjunct from one entire sphere of its own activity: the sustenance given through repetitive labors such as that of the imagination in determinative judgment or of matter when it grows, reproduces and heals. The furthering of the movement forth (*weiterschreiten im Fortschreiten*) thus hits upon paradoxes similar to those presented by the human apprehension of natural organisms. For this, the human animal, more than *Naturzweck*, but also one, will have to come in its origins to reach the ends it sets itself, that is, to heautonomously produce them *into* time.[86] Under these conditions, it would either have to fly free of its tie to reproduction or appear as temporarily disjunctive from itself, that is, as the originator of causal chains within given forms of causation. This kind of embodied moral agent would have to realize itself through activity which would only retrospectively (*nachträglich*) assure the origins of its ends; pointing forward and concluding at once. Further, the kind of reasoner who generates time in acts of apprehension would have to enter time *collectively* and self-constitute *morally-historically*.[87] In some sense, then, it is the reader who

---

86 In her lectures Arendt consistently asserts that of the three great questions motivating the critique, "none of [them] concerns man as a *zoon politikon*, a political being" nor do the questions offer an account of action: publicity steps in the place of action. Hannah Arendt, *Lectures on Kant's Political Philosophy*, ed. Ronald Beiner (Chicago: Chicago University Press, 1982). This attribute of Kant's critical philosophy leads Goetschel to take another step and assert: "… Kant defines reason as nothing other than universal reason, envisioned as the chorus of the voices of 'everybody.' His epistemological model thus is intrinsically political." (*Constituting Critique*, 5)

87 Though such a possibility is directly negated in his following work *Die Religion innerhalb der Grenzen der bloßen Vernunft*, Förster's arguments concerning the *Opus posthumum* leave room to hope that Kant may not have held inflexibly to the position he takes in that work that only God can bring about the moral commonwealth. To quote Förster: "On the one hand, we cannot comprehend a free interference by an extraworldly substance with the law-governed course of nature: 'No miracles take place in the corporeal world,' Kant pronounced in an earlier passage of the *Opus posthumum*, and also in the so called 'Kiesewetter

must vitiate the gap. But how shall she do this alone? Like Shelley's novel, Kant's *Critique of Judgment* leaves the frame open and releases the work to its *readers*.

Aufsätze' (21:439.18; 18:320-22). On the other hand, God cannot realize what is morally good directly through men. God can *demand* that we act morally but *cannot make* us do so. 'The question whether God could not give man a better will would amount to this: that he should make it the case that [man] wills what he does not will.' And 'It is not even in the divine power to make a morally good man (to make him morally good): He must do it himself.' (21:37, 83, Op. 239, 249)." (*Kant's Final Synthesis*, 145)

Chapter Three

Kleist's *Penthesilea, Ein Trauerspiel*

They cross it with the trail of their names and are soon gone. Every time the writer sets down a word, he must fight to win them back. The mercurial quality that heralds their appearance is token also of their evanescence. It wasn't always thus. At least not so long as we had a liturgy. That weave of word and gesture, that aura of controlled destruction, that use of certain materials rather than others: this gratified the gods so long as men chose to turn to them. After which, like windblown scraps in an abandoned encampment, all that was left were the stories that every ritual gesture implied. Uprooted from their soil and exposed, in the vibration of the word, to the harsh light of day, they frequently seemed idle and impudent. Everything ends up as history of literature.
– *Roberto Calasso,* "The Pagan School"

11. Archäologischer Einwand.
Aber der Leib war Erz des Achill! Der Tochter des Ares
Geb' ich zum essen, beim Styx, nichts als die Ferse nur
preis.
– Heinrich von Kleist, *Phöbus Fragmente*

The peculiar autonomy of aesthetic imagination, with its subterranean connections to the material form of living entities, yielded a series of contradictions for Kant's critique: the most general and formal became "raw substrate," an action in time drew its resource from a reserve beyond time, a solitary subject acceded to a collectivity through reflection alone. The desire to bring some, if only obliquely demonstrable, necessity to the curious terrain of reflective judgment entailed a highly versatile conception of a totality, which though to some extent groundless, could afford a glimpse of concept-formation as itself inherently productive of its own grounding, its own lawfulness. Further, in the dynamic realtion between the ultimate constitution of objects and the activity of such constitution, a formal definition of culture emerged which presented the properly cultural historical as generative of its own content *as* form. In the semantic field which stretches between *Zweck* and *tauglich* – the human as *end* or simply *suitable* or *fit* – the force of the "spontaneity of a cause in freedom" stuttered off in analogies of scale, totalities which mirror, but which also empty the possibility of the encounter with human and cultural plurality as itself a matter of form.

Heinrich von Kleist's *Penthesilea, ein Trauerspiel* rounds on such a wish for an ultimate univocality and presents his readers and audience with a dilemma of staging which, like Kant's *Critique of Judgment*, might catch out the simultaneously autonomous and mechanical function of imagination in its generation of conceptual forms. In the logic of its composition, however, *Penthesilea* will not rest with the fiction of the solitary subject occupied solely by generative acts of self-determination but introduces the pulse of conflict, dialogue, encounter as the setting for any such scene of judgment. *Penthesilea* treats of words caught in the tension and torque of the context in which they are exchanged and the Kleistian theatrical word achieves a doubling of space at the juncture between the generative capacity and destructive force of language as it makes and remakes a world onstage.

Kleist's *Trauerspiel* resists summary retelling, because the status of any given action in it remains open to dispute – riven and multiple at the same time. Like Shelley's daemon who springs directly forth from philosophy with an autobiography which reads like an 18th-century philosophical fiction, Kleist's *Penthesilea* also stages the narration of an origin story as an event that takes place in the context of a dialogue where both persuasion and force are in play. At the center of Kleist's *Trauerspiel*, Penthesilea narrates the origin of her "culture" *twice* and that telling prepares the ground for the mournful and violent doublings of interpretation that ensue. In this sense both Kleist and Shelley recode the 18th-century genre of the speculative origin story as itself an act within history, and which – in keeping with the paradoxes of enlightened historical action presented in Kant's essay on the Enlightenment – constitutes a point of origin in its own right.

The Weimar Classical stage, generally understood to be comprised of the dogma and productions of Schiller and Goethe between 1795-1805, and to which Kleist arguably made a contribution with his *Penthesilea*, had assumed many of the enlightenment themes of the problem of tracing culture's threshold. In its attempt to indicate the origins of a hopefully renewed humanity sitting right there in the audience, it offered a reflection upon its ancestry that could itself constitute a site of cultural inception, a national beginning.[1] In their own theorization of how the theater might simultaneously bind and unleash the powers of the imagination, Goethe and Schiller join the discussions of the relay between general and particular, ideal and real and collective acts of self-constitution, by presenting a form of theatrical ideality that could harmonize the enlightenment doubles we have been considering so far – the moral and the natural, the man and the citizen, the prototype and the instance – though they also notably add to this series the dyad of the sister and the subject. Kleist's *Penthesilea, Ein Trauerspiel* also touches on these questions, though in Kleist's theater, every double runs the risk of encountering its counterpart as other and colliding with it. *Penthesilea* addresses the twining of myth with history on a new national German stage and projects for literary self-understanding based on the revisitation of Greek antiquity.[2] His drama stages the moment of ethnographic encounter between a literary tradition and its interrogation of the "origin" of culture. Following too closely the letter of the law, Kleist radically recasts the *active* principle of ideality in Weimar Classicism as the grounds for an experiment in representation more akin to science fiction than Neoclassicism.[3]

The Penthesilea Effect

Penthesilea moves with Dr. Frankenstein's daemon at high speed in imaginary realms either side of the "human." The eponymous heroine, barely glimpsed for the first five scenes of the play – during which she is described as coursing around the perimeter of the stage with the force and speed of a hurricane – taxes the capacities of representation. Like Frankenstein's daemon she is "given," but there is no concept for her. In Odysseus' well-known and oft-cited description, she escapes designation in terms of the opposition force/resistance ("So viel ich weiß, gibt es in der

---

1 For a helpful introduction to Weimar Classicism see Norbert Oellers and Robert Steegers, eds., *Treffpunkt Weimar* (Stuttgart: Reclam, 1999), 124-92.

2 For a discussion of the history of Enlightenment and the study of antiquity stretching from Petrarch through Kleist's time and beyond, see Peter Gay's *The Enlightenment.* Peter Gay, *The Enlightenment: The Rise of Modern Paganism* (New York: W.W. Norton & Co., 1995), vol. 1 and 2.

3 See Slavoj Zizek and his designation of Kleist as a member of the line of "truly subversive authors": Not "transgressors à la Sade but those (from Pascal through Kleist to Brecht's learning plays) who belong to the overconformist line: Authors who subvert the ruling ideology by taking it more literally than it is ready to take itself." Slavoj Zizek, "Why Does the Law Need an Obscene Supplement?" in *Law and The Postmodern Mind: Essays on Psychoanalysis and Jurisprudence*, ed. Peter Goodrich and David Gray Carlson (Ann Arbor, University of Michigan Press, 1998), 75.

Natur/Kraft bloß und ihren Widerstand, nichts Drittes") [1.125-126][4] "I thought till now that Nature knows but force/And counterforce, and no third power besides."[5] Penthesilea can't be pinned down, and in some sense the *Trauerspiel* is organized around her indefinability and the corollary attempt to claim or anchor it through acts of negation and affirmation on the part of other players on the stage.

Penthesilea describes an arc of motion; she appears and reappears in a shifting, flexible range of alternating registers touched upon by the desire to signify her – the persistent attempt to catch her in simile. The figure of the Amazon queen is also simultaneously overburdened with the tokens of particular attributes, distinguishing marks of every turn: her participation in an alien creed and her non-participation in that creed, her status as woman and her status as the other or the exceeder of woman, her role as leader (*Herrscherin*) and as pariah. Figured as both the movement of desire and as the tree blasted and uprooted by it, the virtuosity of Penthesilea spans her participation in an animal resource and urgency as well as a heroic force.

---

4 Heinrich von Kleist, *Sämtliche Werke und Briefe*, vol. 2, ed. Hans Rudolf Barth et al. (Frankfurt am Main: Deutscher Klassiker Verlag, 1987), 143-256. Citations are provided with line numbers so that my reading may be followed with any numbered edition. Walter Müller-Seidel has commented on Kleist's "nichts Drittes" in his chapter "Kleists *Penthesilea* im Kontext der deutschen Klassik." He argues that for Kleist the well-worn idealist concept of "the third" withdraws from the concept of opposition thesis/antithesis ("Das Dritte ist für Kleist jener Bereich, der sich den Vorstellungen entzieht, in denen Satz und Gegensatz, Teil und Gegenteil gelten"). (Walter Müller-Seidel, *Die Geschichtlichkeit der deutschen Klassik: Literatur und Denkformen um 1800* [Stuttgart: Metzlersche Verlagsbuchhandlung, 1983], 216). It is important to recall that Odysseus effectively calls the Amazons not "the third" but "nothing third" (the line also does not run "kein Drittes," using the negation of the accusative or direct object but rather "nichts Drittes" in the nominative through apposition). Carol Jacobs makes the point that Odysseus produces his own slip of the tongue: "Odysseus may not be, as Penthesilea will put it later, 'master of the rash lip.' Just when he asserts that water cannot act as fire, Odysseus speaks of fire rather than water: 'What puts out the glow of fire.' Water and fire, it seems, can only be named by way of their opposites – in the very moment of insisting that this is what they are not. Still, although the gesture may be confusing, when the teetertotter of rhetorical substitution stops, one can see that the logic of the statement holds (Carol Jacobs, *Uncontainable Romanticism: Shelley, Brontë, Kleist* [Baltimore: Johns Hopkins University Press, 1989], 92-93). Here are the lines in question: "Was Glut des Feuers löscht, löst Wasser siedend/Zu dampf nicht auf und umgekehrt…" [1.127-128]. Further, Kleist has laced the entire verse with steam.

5 Heinrich von Kleist, *Penthesilea: A Tragic Drama*, trans. Joel Agee (Harper Collins Publishers, 1998), 8. Henceforth pages numbers to this translation will be provided in parentheses and I will note any alterations to Agee's translations.

Penthesilea also meddles with tradition by presenting the performative speaker[6] *par excellence*, what Gabrielle Brandstetter and Gerhard Neumann have termed "inverted prosopopoeia ... not the lending of a face, voice and living form to one dead, but rather the inverse, the metamorphosis of the living into the dead."[7] Whereas Frankenstein's daemon came alive and spoke, Penthesilea speaks herself dead with a fatal word of comparison "so" (the speech: "So! So! So! So! Und wieder! – Nun ist's gut," [148] which might also be rendered "Thus! Thus! Thus! Thus! and Again! – Now it's good." Or "Like this! Like this! Like this!...) and a gesture. In this she must be recognized as a "performative speaker" in a complex way, for it is not that she says "I die" as one might say "I marry," but she says "thus" having first forged in her previous words the image of a dagger.[8] While the difficult-to-locate Penthesilea may challenge the limits of theatrical representation in the first scenes of the play, in the last she abuses the possibilities of theatrical illusion to the fullest: her verbally effectuated suicide is a species of *deus ex machina* of the most startling kind. Despite our persistent fascination with its implications, the theater that stages Kleist's *Penthesilea* would have us believe that the transubstantiation of words into material things has been wrought. But, after all, it is a play, and rarely has anyone died on stage through more than a gesture.

At the very least we can say that Kleist's staging of the play forgoes the stage prop for the dagger in this scene, or substitutes words in the place of the object. In another sense, however, the field of forces which constitutes Penthesilea's demise defies unequivocal explanation. To take the words used by Jean-Pierre Vernant in describing the tragic subject:

---

6 For a definition of "performative speech" see J. L. Austin, *How to Do Things with Words* (Cambridge: Harvard University Press, 1975), 4-11. See Derrida on the problem of maintaining the distinction between *performative* and *constative*. Jacques Derrida, "Déclarations d'indépendence" in *Otobiographies: l'enseignement de Nietzsche et la politique du nom propre* (Paris: Gallimard, 1984), 19-20. See Butler on the subversive potential of performativity as well as an expansion of what the category could designate. Judith Butler, *Gender Trouble: Feminism and the Subversion of Identity* (New York: Routledge, 2006), 175-203.

7 Gabrielle Brandstetter and Gerhard Neumann, "Opferfest – Sacre du Printemps," in *Konflikt, Grenze, Dialog: Kulturkontrastive und interdisziplinäre Textzugänge* (Frankfurt am Main: Peter Lang, 1997), 116-117: Brandstetter and Neumann rely here on Hillis Miller's articulation of the concept of prosopopoeia in *Versions of Pygmalion* (Cambridge: Harvard University Press, 1990).

8 In her reading of the play, Carol Jacobs regards this scene as demonstrative of a fatal collapse between words and deeds: "There is no temporal or spatial rift between words and deeds" (Jacobs, *Uncontainable Romanticism*, 113). Jacobs argues: "The passage is at once the most daring of metaphorical conceits and, if we are to judge by the success of her fall ('She falls and dies'), language as its own absolute, immediate realization" (Ibid., 114). I would add to this a consideration of the staging of the act somewhere between the stage presence of words, bodies and things in Kleist's peculiar form of theater.

"...within the space of the stage and the framework of tragic representation, the hero is no longer put forward as a model, as he used to be in epic and in lyric poetry. Now he has become a problem ... ."[9] By the end of the play – in inverse direction to Frankenstein's daemon – Penthesilea is unnamed by the phrase, "the answer to the gruesome riddle" (*das Wort des Greuelrätsels*) and the problem encompassed by *Penthesilea* reflects as much on the determination of the "human" as it does on representation.[10]

If, around 1800, tragedy is understood to encapsulate the universally human at culture's threshold, Kleist's *Penthesilea* seems to recognize the potential uses implied by the recourse to tragedy as demarcating the line between literary culture and its antecedents.[11] As cultural artifact, tragedy gradually comes to be regarded over the course of the nineteenth century as both treating this issue and performing it.[12] Kleist's *Trauerspiel*, specifically naming itself through reference to its Baroque and not its classical ancestor, reflects critically upon this possibility. When Penthesilea springs

9 Jean-Pierre Vernant and Pierre Vidal-Naquet, *Myth and Tragedy in Ancient Greece* (New York: Zone Books, 1988), 242.

10 On the issue of the limits of theatrical representation and Kleist's *Penthesilea* one can look to two hundred years of comment on the problem beginning with Goethe's reservations (*Lebensspuren*, No. 224). *Heinrich von Kleists Lebensspuren Dokumente und Berichte der Zeitgenossen*, ed. Helmut Semdner (Munich: Hanser, 1996). Detlev von Liliencorn satirized the idea of staging the piece in 1885: "Elephanten werden vorgeführt!" (*Nachruhm,* 661) in much the same vein as Kleist's contemporary Karl August Böttiger in 1808 (*Lebensspuren* Nr. 225a). *Heinrich von Kleists Nachruhm: Eine Wirkungsgeschichte in Dokumente* (Munich: Hanser, 1996). See also the following which all appear in *Kleist Jahrbuch 2001* (Stuttgart: Verlag J. B. Metzler, 2001): Manfred Schneider, "Die Welt im Ausnahmezustand," 104-119; Alexander Kosenina, "Will er 'auf ein Theater warten, welches da kommen soll?,'" 38-54; and Hans-Thies Lehmann, "Kleist/Versionen" also in *Kleist Jahrbuch 2001*, 89-103.

11 For a compelling discussion of the long Antigone tradition in Western philosophy and psychoanalysis, especially in terms of the question of 'culture's threshold,' see Judith Butler, *Antigone's Claim: Kinship between Life and Death* (New York: Columbia University Press, 2002).

12 See Peter Szondi's *An Essay on the Tragic* for a discussion of the emergence of a "philosophy of the tragic" in distinction to a "historical poetics of tragedy." Szondi writes, "By interpreting the tragic process as the self-division and self-reconciliation of the ethical nature, Hegel makes his dialectical structure immediately apparent for the first time. ... the tragic and the dialectic coincide." Peter Szondi, *An Essay on the Tragic*, trans. Paul Fleming (Stanford: Stanford University Press, 2002), 16-17. For Hegel on Antigone see §451-452, §457, §470-471 in *The Phenomenology of Spirit* and §108, §140-142 in *The Philosophy of Right.* Between Goethe's treatment of the Iphigenia material to approach the ethos of the universal condition of 'woman' and Hegel's treatment of Antigone as representing the special status of the sister – "intuitive awareness of the Ethical" – which facilitates a transition between forms of legal universality, the sister figure from tragedy powerfully contributes to the staging of a historical development and offers the limit-case for different forms of political and cultural self-awareness. Neither a brother's sister nor a bride, Kleist's Penthesilea moves at a marked remove from these exemplary figures.

"like lightening" between the Greek and Trojan troops, she may also be breaking up a Weimar performance. It is possible that the mythology he proposes to reinvent derives less from the Ancient Greeks than the enlightened mythology of cultural transition they were coming to inform. Goethe's *Iphigenie auf Tauris* opens up the literary-philosophical *Spannungsfeld* within which Kleist's phantasmatic troops of Amazons take the stage. If there is a "classical" text that forms Kleist's intertext for *Penthesilea*, then it must be this Iphigenie of Goethe, whose heart mirrors the will of the gods and whose *will* transforms the historical-cultural practices of her "barbaric" host. Kleist seems to have recognized the informant role ancient tragedy was coming to play for literature and to have *staged* the scene of this exchange between literary inheritor and culturally *emergent* ancestor. In this, Kleist's negotiation of the distinctions key to the theatrical principles of Weimar also points to the ethical significance of every interpretive act.

Weimar Classicism and the Double: The Speaking Body on Stage

In a prose piece from 1803 written as a companion to *Die Braut von Messina* and published in *Die Horen*, "Über den Gebrauch des Chors in der Tragödie," Schiller attributes remarkable synthetic powers to the "art theater" (*Kunsttheater*).

> Wie aber nun die Kunst zugleich ganz ideell und doch im tiefsten Sinne reell sein – wie das Wirkliche ganz verlassen und doch aufs genauste mit den Natur übereinstimmen soll und kann, das ist's, was wenige fassen, was die Ansicht poetischer und plastischer Werke so schielend macht, weil beide Forderungen einander im gemeinen Urteil geradezu aufzuheben scheinen.
>
> Auch begegnet es gewöhnlich, daß man das eine mit Aufopferung des andern zu erreichen sucht und eben deswegen beides verfehlt. (283)
>
> But how art can and shall be at once ideal and yet in the profoundest sense real – how it can and shall totally abandon actuality and at the same time conform exactly to nature – this is what few people understand, this is what makes the view of poetic and plastic works so ambiguous, because the two demands seem to cancel each other completely out in the general opinion.
>
> It usually happens, moreover, that people try to achieve the one at the sacrifice of the other and by so doing miss both.[13]

13 Friedrich Schiller, "On the Use of the Chorus in Tragedy" in *The Bride of Messina, William Tell, Demetrius*, trans. Charles E Passage (New York: Frederick Ungar Publishing, 1962), 5.

Here, in Kantian vein, "nature" becomes a term to be subtly differentiated from the "real" (*das Wirkliche*). Nature is an idea, and interestingly, as an idea, it underwrites the project of a certain conception of theater.

> Phantastische Gebilde willkürlich aneinander reihen, heißt nicht ins Ideale gehen, und das Wirkliche nachahmend wieder bringen, heißt nicht die Natur darstellen. Beide Forderungen stehen so wenig im Widerspruch mit einander, daß sie vielmehr – eine und dieselbe sind; daß die Kunst nur dadurch wahr ist, daß sie das Wirkliche ganz verläßt und rein ideell wird. Die Natur selbst ist nur eine Idee des Geistes, die nie in die Sinne fällt. Unter der Decke der Erscheinungen liegt sie, aber sie selbst kommt niemals zur Erscheinung. Bloß der Kunst des Ideals ist es verliehen, oder vielmehr aufgegeben, diesen Geist des Alls zu ergreifen und in einer körperlichen Form zu binden ... Es ergibt sich daraus von selbst, daß der Künstler kein einziges Element aus der Wirklichkeit brauchen kann, wie er es findet, daß sein Werk in allen seinen Teilen ideell sein muß, wenn es als ein Ganzes Realität haben und mit der Natur übereinstimmen soll. (284)

> Arbitrary lining up of fantastic pictures one after another is not penetrating into the ideal, and imitative reproduction of actuality is not portrayal of Nature. The two claims contradict each other so little that they are really one and the same, namely that art is true only as it abandons actuality altogether and becomes purely ideal. Nature itself is only an idea of the spirit, an idea which never comes to sensory perception. It lies beneath the veil of phenomenon. Only to the art of the ideal is it vouchsafed, or rather enjoined as an obligation, to grasp this spirit of the universe and to encompass it within a corporeal form ... It follows, then, that the artist cannot use a single element from actuality as he finds it, that his work must be ideal in *all* its parts if it is to have reality as a whole and be in consonance with Nature.[14]

"Nature" is the term for the non-actual, which steers a course between the fantastic and the contingent and thereby allows for the reconciliation of the ideal with the real. In a certain sense, it is the *talk* of nature and, more importantly, the impossibility of its direct cognition, that makes of "nature" precisely that term that exposes the possibility of this reconciliation. Nature, in this context, is an *example* of the harmonizing and rubricating activity of an organizing principle that both anchors and transcends the vagaries of the actual. Both narrative and theatrical *Darstellung* are measured against the standard of the "whole" – the formal principle that serves to distinguish between the actual and the true. Generating coherent wholes poses the prime activity of the artist who deploys this formal criterion to impart necessity to the composition, and perhaps also the reception, of the artwork. When we consider that nature is an "idea" – and the reader must be vigilant in remembering this, for it demands an active re-

14 Ibid., 6.

casting of a more common usage of the word – the most remarkable result is that we are not, in fact, grappling with a difficult paradox. The theater is active in the process of making, of corroborating, of aiding and abetting an idea. It is not so much a question of the paradoxical inversion that theatrical presentations seem more real the more unreal they are, but rather that the theater actively mimics not reality but ideation. Brought before not only the senses but also *the imagination* and through the "schaffende Gewalt" of the senses, the ideal becomes the generative resource that is annexed to a larger process of necessity-building. In its artificing, tragedy communicates with the imagination via the senses and the production, by this definition, is "non-versimilar" though it is also deeply "true." Without this regulatory operation of the idea nothing can be built or founded in the mind (*Gemüt*).

> Wem hingegen zwar eine rege Phantasie, aber ohne Gemüt und Charakter zu teil geworden, der wird sich um keine Wahrheit bekümmern, sondern mit dem Weltstoff nur spielen, nur durch phantastische und bizarre Kombinationen zu überraschen suchen und wie sein ganzes Tun nur Schaum und Schein ist, so wird er zwar für den Augenblick unterhalten, aber im Gemüt nichts erbauen und begründen. (284)

> On the other hand, one endowed with a lively fantasy but without soul and character, will not be worried about any truth but will merely play with the world-material, will try merely to surprise us with fantastic and bizarre combinations, and, since his whole activity is only froth and illution, he will entertain us for the moment but he will not found and construct anything in our spirits.[15]

Here we are witness to a requirement laid upon the activities of the imagination which is made in the name of laying foundations. One might further reflect that the particular penchant of Schiller's explicitly Kantian aesthetics need not necessarily constitute the sole option for engaging the constructive capacity of the imaginative faculty. One might alternately recall the preemptive apology for the novel *Frankenstein* (attributed to P. B. Shelley) and its unnamed fabrication, Dr. Frankenstein's monster.

> [H]owever impossible as a physical fact, [it] affords a point of view to the imagination for the delineating of human passions more comprehensive and commanding than any which the *ordinary relations of existing events* can yield.[16]

On the one hand, this passage would seem to be very much in the spirit of Schiller's goals for the theater. On the other, the monster to which it refers is indisputably *unnatural* both as a composite body and as a non-

15 Ibid., 5-6.

16 Shelley, *Frankenstein,* 7.

harmonizing idea. But how is this third term "nature" important for Schiller's conception of theater? These passages on the use of the chorus resonate clearly with the broader discussion concerning the particular and the general that has concerned this study. For Schiller's purposes the chorus presents a welcome interruption of the unfreedom of a too-passional response to events on stage that might be mistaken for "real." The chorus raises the level of the speeches – imparting to them that artistry that Schiller compares to the sculpting of veils, a "*lyrische Prachtgewebe*," (*a lyrical cloth of splendor*) – and provides that the spectators don't lose themselves in the material but float or drift above it. This occurs partly because the chorus serves to separate "reflection" (*Reflexion*) from "action" (*Handlung*).[17] However, in the distance placed between action and reflection we encounter a return of the disavowed term "natural" (*Das Natürliche* as opposed to *Natur*), used earlier in the essay to describe mere mimeticism in theatrical productions.[18] The "natural" is suffered a brief return at the end of the argument, as adjective, when it is asserted that the tragic players "stand on a to some extent natural theater" insofar as they stand before the chorus. The actors

> stehen gewissermaßen schon auf einem natürlichen Theater, weil sie vor Zuschauern sprechen und handeln, und werden eben deswegen desto tauglicher von dem Kunst-Theater zu einem Publikum zu reden. (290)
>
> stand on a natural stage because they speak and act before spectators, and by that token they come to speak more becomingly from an artificial stage (*Kunsttheater*) to an audience. (11)

The chorus produces a natural theater within the boundaries of the aesthetically distanced classical stage. These figures therefore speak before both a "natural" (that is, "on-stage") public and a secondary "off-stage" public. The curious tension that arises between the body and the voice of these actors when on stage is emphasized in the passage below by the parallel position of the two verbal constructions of "to bind in a physical (bodily) form" and "pronounce."

> [D]enn sie [tragischen Personen] sind keine wirkliche Wesen, die bloß der Gewalt des Moments gehorchen, und bloß ein Individuum darstellen, sondern ideale Personen und Repräsentanten ihrer Gattung, die das Tiefe der Menschheit aussprechen. (290)

---

17 "Der Chor reinigt also das tragische Gedicht, indem er die Reflexion von der Handlung absondert, und eben durch diese Absonderung sie selbst mit poetischer Kraft ausrüstet" (Schiller, "Über den Gebrauch des Chors," 288).

18 "Auch hier hatte man lange und hat noch jetzt mit dem gemeinen Begriff des Natürlichen zu kämpfen, welcher alle Poesie and Kunst geradezu aufhebt und vernichtet" (Ibid., 284-85).

> The tragic persons likewise have need of this respite, this calm, to collect themselves, for they are not real beings that merely obey the force of the moment and represent mere individuals, but ideal personages and representatives of their class, who pronounce upon the profound in mankind.[19]

They do not represent individuals but embody genres (*Gattungen:* species, genres, genders). This is the process described in a long passage cited above by which the art of the ideal "binds the spirit of the totality (*Geist des Alls*) in a physical form." As embodied general or ideal forms, these tragic persons pronounce/embody the "depth" of humanity. Nonetheless they do work with the imagination via the senses. One might say that they are concrete but not particular.

The chorus as witness restrains its outbursts of passion and motivates the reflectiveness (*Besonnenheit*) with which these genre-figures act. The talking weaves of Schiller's stage return original and naive motifs to the theater. In so doing, they rely on the chorus' destruction of everything that resists poetry, and they give an immediate general expression to forms of social being which no longer exist. In this sense, their ideality is also notably historically and culturally inflected.

> Der Palast der Könige ist jetzt geschlossen, die Gerichte haben sich von den Toren der Städte in das Innere der Häuser zurückgezogen, die Schrift hat das lebendige Wort verdrängt, das Volk selbst, die sinnlich lebendige Masse, ist, wo sie nicht als rohe Gewalt wirkt, zum Staat, folglich zu einem abgezogenen Begriff geworden, die Götter sind in die Brust des Menschen zurückgekehrt. Der Dichter muß die Paläste wieder auftun, er muß die Gerichte unter freien Himmel herausführen, er muß die Götter wieder aufstellen, er muß alles Unmittelbare, das durch die künstliche Einrichtung des wirklichen Lebens aufgehoben ist, wieder herstellen, und alles künstliche Machwerk an dem Menschen und um denselben, das die Erscheinung seiner innern Natur und seines ursprünglichen Charakters hindert, wie der Bildhauer die modernen Gewänder, abwerfen, und von allen äußern Umgebungen desselben nichts aufnehmen, als was die höchste der Formen, die menschliche, sichtbar macht. (286-87)

> The palace of the kings is now closed; the judges have retreated from the gates of the city to the interiors of houses; the letter has crowded out the living word; the people themselves, that materially living mass, has become the state, – unless it is acting as raw force, – and hence has become an abstract principle; and the gods have returned to the bosoms of men. The poet must reopen the palaces, he must once again bring the judges forth beneath the open skies, he must establish the gods anew, he must restore everything that is direct and which has been abolished by the artificial arrangements of actual life, he must cast off all artificial contrivances in man and around which hinder the manifestation of his inner nature and his original character, just as

19 Ibid., 11.

> sculptors cast away modern garments and accept nothing of all external surroundings except what renders visible the highest of forms, – human form.[20]

Here Schiller synchronizes and makes apposite a string of differentiated losses and relatively unspecified historical developments: a shift away from regal ceremony, the withdrawal behind doors of tribunals, the increasing primacy of literacy through the printing press, the reduction of the masses to the representative abstraction of the state (unless they break forth into brute force), and finally, the re-internalization of the gods in the human "breast." The body of the tragic performer, however, reverses these losses with his or her particular form of stage presence and reconcretizes civic life.

In Schiller's theorization of the chorus, the question of a speaking, sensual presence brought to stand in for the realities of a state legislation withdrawn behind doors is both sublimated and foregrounded. The idealized mythic body on the stage encodes this history at the same time that it works to reconcile it through the active effects of the body's presence on the stage. The question of such *speaking* presences and the reinternalization of the gods in the human breast leads us directly to Goethe's *Iphigenie auf Tauris*, in which the simultaneously lost and present body of Agamemnon's daughter-sacrifice stands and speaks. In her opening lines she *presents* her absence by tracing the split between her social and material being. Let us turn now to Iphigenie.

Iphigenie auf Tauris

The play begins with Iphigenie, alone on stage, emphasizing a series of split modes of being, which, meanwhile, she univocally comprises in her person. The audience witnesses her at the scene of the exile to which she was "spirited" away. She is "bewahrt verborgen" (*preserved hidden*) as she stands on stage, saying: "Doch immer bin ich, wie im ersten fremd" (*Indeed, I remain, as from the first, alien/foreign*) (*I.i.7-9*).[21] She stands there against the emptiness of exile she conjures in her words, both scenically and in terms of her self-understanding. "Und an dem Ufer steh ich lange Tage…" (*And on the shore I stand for long days*) (*I.i.11*). Finally, at the end of her first speech she names her life thus delivered the "second death" pleading with the goddess Diana: "Und rette mich, die du vom Tod errettet,/Auch von dem Leben hier, dem zweiten Tod!" (*And save me, whom you saved from death/Also from life here, from the second death!*) (*I.2.52-53*).

---

20 Ibid., 8.

21 Johann Wolfgang von Goethe, *Sämtliche Werke*, vol. 5, ed. Peter Huber (Frankfurt am Main: Deutscher Klassiker Verlag, 1988), 553-620. All lines numbers cited parenthetically.

In this active presencing of absences in Iphigenie's opening speech the tension between her "*Zustand*" (circumstance) and her *Herkunft/Zukunft* (fate)[22] drives the significance of her words. The first death of the mythical sacrifice, the bind she was in until she was transported away from the "sanften Bänden" (*gentle ties to kith and kin*) has given way to her surprisingly unexpected summation of the problem: "Ich rechne mit den Göttern nicht; allein/Der Frauen Zustand ist beklagenswert" (*I do not argue with the gods, only/The condition of women is lamentable*) (*I.i.23-24*). This last "-wert" falls with a wooden finality in the last iamb; the whole melodic *enchaînement* that has flowed through the preceding lines drops to stillness. This coming to rest on "-wert" marks the transition to the lament, not of her tragic condition but of her general position (*Zustand*) qua *woman*. The opening monologue sets the stage for Iphigenie's ensuing series of speeches that culminate in the acknowledgment that all she has *is* words. "Ich habe nichts als Worte…"

Laß ab! Beschönige nicht die Gewalt,
Die sich der Schwachheit eines Weibes freut.
Ich bin so freigeboren als ein Mann.
Stünd' Agammemnons Sohn dir gegenüber
Und du verlangtest, was sich nicht gebührt:
So hat auch *er* ein Schwert und einen Arm,
Die Rechte seines Busens zu verteid'gen.
Ich habe nichts als Worte, und es ziemt
Dem edlen Mann, der Frauen Wort zu achten. (V.3. 1856-1864)

Do not seek to extenuate the harshness
That takes advantage of a woman's weakness.
I am as free-born as a man. And if
The son of Agamemnon stood before you,
And if you asked improper things of him,
He has a sword and has an arm to wield it
In his defense of the rights of his heart.

---

22 For a strong position on the correct understanding of *Mythos* for Goethe's stage, Adorno's Iphigenie essay is of note. "Vom Mythos redet er (Artur Henkel) nicht, wie der schlampige Sprachgebrauch, im Sinn von Gleichnissen für Überzeitliches oder Transzendentes, sondern ähnlich wie Benjamin in dem Traktat über die *Wahlverwandtschaften*, als vom Schuldzusammenhang des Lebendigen, dem Schicksal. Solcher Mythos, gegenwärtige Vorwelt, ist im gesamten Goetheschen Werke vorhanden." "Henkel does not conform to the sloppy practice of speaking about myth as a figure for something supratemporal or transcendental: rather, as Benjamin does in the tractatus of Goethe's *Elective Affinities*, he speaks of it as the web of guilt in which the living are entangled, as fate. Myth in this sense, a present-day prehistorical world, is present throughout the whole of Goethe's oeuvre." (Theodor Adorno, "Zum Klassizismus von Goethe's Iphigenie," in *Noten zur Literatur* (Frankfurt am Main: Suhrkamp, 1979). Translated by Shierry Weber Nicholsen under the title *Notes to Literature* (New York: Columbia University Press, 1992), 153-154.

But I have only words, and it beseems
A noble man to value women's words.[23]

If one were to look for the vestige of myth at the conclusion of *Iphigenie auf Tauris*, it might well reside in the utopian transfer of universal-as-masculine to universal-as-feminine undertaken in the passage cited above. Iphigenie herein becomes the representative of the rights-seeking community (Mileans) *par excellence* by dint of her relative (physical) impuissance and her invocation of it in this speech. She argues for her rights on the strength of her eloquence alone, all the time pointing to the use of force requisite to the assurance of them. In this manner the "Enlightenment for woman" slips a *new myth* in with classical garb. Notably, the rights thus argued for are those particularized in the "breast" of the individual, though they are simultaneously generalized as the circumstance of women (*Frauenzustand*). From the site of the body rescued from its status as sacrificial victim, Iphigenie speaks herself in and out of existence – first eliding her social existence and then becoming the agent of it – always operating from the empty grounds and hollow tones of the unanswering waves on the shore, the second death, which do ultimately bring her Orestes and allow her to save the brother in the name of the father.[24]

When Goethe's Iphigenie splits and doubles herself by speaking for speech she also comes to house in her one body the dynamic tension between Athena and the chorus of Eumenides which closes Aeschylus' treatment of the house of Tantalus myth. "Plunge beneath the ground"

23 Johann Wolfgang von Goethe, *Goethe's Plays*, trans. Charles E. Passage (New York: Frederick Ungar Publishing Co., 1980), 469-70.

24 René Girard makes the point in *Violence and the Sacred* that: "It is clearly legitimate to define the difference between sacrificable and nonsacrificable individuals in terms of their degree of integration, but such a definition is not yet sufficient. In many cultures women are never, or rarely, selected as sacrificial victims. There may be a simple explanation for this fact. The married woman retains her ties with her parents' clan after she has become in some respects the property of her husband and his family. To kill her would be to run the risk of one of the two groups' interpreting her sacrifice as an act of murder committing it to a reciprocal act of revenge" (Rene Girard, *Violence and the Sacred*, trans. Patrick Gregory [Baltimore: Johns Hopkins University Press, 1977], 13). Clytaemnestra with her act of vengeance refuses Agammemnon's property in Iphigenie. This is the same sacrifice that Iphigenie is busy reworking and revitalizing on Goethe's stage. Goethe's Iphigenie forgets Clytaemnestra – Orestes asks, "Und fürchtest du für Klytaemestra nichts?" ("Do you not fear for Clytaemnestra?) – and his sister is confronted with the following riddle: she did not spill her own blood but her own blood gave her death ("doch ihr eigen Blut gab ihr Tod"). One result of Clytaemnestra's act, however, is that Iphigenie finds herself without husband or father: "Von Jugend auf habe ich gelernt gehorchen,/Erst meinen Eltern und denn einer Gottheit./Und folgsam fühlt' ich immer meine Seele,/Am schönsten frei, allein dem harten Worte/Dem rauhen Ausspruch eines Mannes mich/zu fügen, lernt ich weder dort noch hier" (V.3.1825-1831).

Athena cries to the chorus of Eumenides. Beneath the ground they are well installed as the angry engine underneath the Parthenon – relegated there by Athena's tie-breaking vote and arts of persuasion – where they comprise a contained survival of the old rule of vengeance as safeguard against further outbreak of civil strife.[25] I recall the denouement of the *Oresteia* in order to bring the older version of Iphigenie's sacrifice into relief and to suggest that there exist some survivals of this alternate tradition in Goethe's treatment of the Tauris material (though compressed into the single figure of Iphigenie). From her self-avowed status within a "second death" Goethe's Iphigenie preserves, within the scope of her one dramatic person, the act of violence that founds the law outside the law, while simultaneously inhabiting the position from which the (new) law's enunciation is performed.[26]

Goethe's *Iphigenie* doesn't spring from her father's head but comes to life with his sacrificial blow – but only in the lapse, the caesura, the second death of her first life's sublimation in Tauris. This is the mode of Iphigenie's form of reconciliation. Her words move in this gap and suture it with the generative stage presence of her coming-to-stand-to-speak – simultaneously incorporating the sacrificed and the non-yet living, that double terrain, which brackets the incredible action of her *presence* on stage according to the theatrical precepts of Weimar Classicism. How are we to construe the relationship between the body and the voice on stage within this context? Let us turn now to the explicit exposition of these precepts coauthored by Goethe and Schiller from the stronghold of their collaboration.[27]

---

25 In the Aulis tradition, Iphigenia's sacrifice is achieved, and her death makes up one link in the chain of retribution stretching from father, mother almost to brother before being legislated to a stop by Athena's deciding vote. The compensation offered the Eumenides is that they will protect the perpetuity of the new, non-retributive order of law from underground, from their base under the Parthenon. Thus the past of blood retribution both founds and haunts the newer order. In Goethe's treatment of the Tauris material, when Iphigenie is saved, spared the sacrifice, it is she who becomes the agent of reconciliation who protects her brother in Athena's place.

26 See Walter Benjamin, "A Critique of Violence," in *Reflections: Essays Aphorisms, Autobiographical Writings* (New York: Harcourt Brace Jovanovich, 1978), and Jacques Derrida, "Force of Law," in *Deconstruction and the Possibility of Justice*, eds. Drucilla Cornell et al. (New York: Routledge, 1992).

27 Schiller's "Über den Gebrauch des Chors in der Tragödie" – contrary to Adorno's ceaselessly inveighing remarks – could be argued to respond to Goethe's project with *Iphigenie*, the first version of which appeared in 1779 and was rewritten several times long prior to Goethe's acquaintance with Schiller.

Über Epische und Dramatische Dichtung

In the letter "Über epische und dramatische Dichtung," Schiller and Goethe set out to define two great classical genres and the laws that govern them.[28] The key points of comparison that structure their difference are the attributes of the speaking body, the parameters of place and movement, the temporal status (i.e., past, present, or future) of the events depicted, and the quality of the audience's participation. Notably, the terms used by Goethe and Schiller to distinguish the two genres do not conform entirely to our understanding of the difference between *bürgerliches Trauerspiel* and *Weimarer Klassik*. That difference is adumbrated in a recent essay by Erika Fischer-Lichte on Kleist's *Prinz Friedrich von Homburg* as the difference between "semiotic bodies" and "aesthetically symbolic" bodies.[29] To summarize: whereas Enlightenment theatrical concepts rely upon a law of analogy to assure that a body's gestural exterior can be decoded as a language through which internal affect is manifest – thereby also cuing the audience's intended affective response – the Classical concept demands that the body of the actor be apprehended symbolically. Referring to Goethe's strict eradication of all "natural" bodily function on stage such as sniffling or spitting, Fischer-Lichte offers the following summary of the difference between the two concepts of the body on stage and the "perceptual models" they call forth.

> Der Körper des Schauspielers [im klassischen Theater] wurde als ein ästhetischer Körper, als Staffage in einem Tableau inszeniert, um dem Zuschauer eine bestimmte Art der Wahrnehmung abzuverlangen, die sich grundlegend von derjenigen im Theater der Aufklärung unterscheidet. Während dort das richtige 'Lesen' der Zeichen, die der Schauspieler mit seinem Körper hervorbrachte, die Einfühlung des Zuschauers in die Figur und sein Mitfühlen erleichterte und beförderte, verlangte Goethes 'harmonisches Ganzes', in das der Schauspieler sich nach malerischen Prinzipien einfügte, dem Zuschauer ästhetische Distanz ab, d.h. er sollte die Bilder und Vorgänge auf der Bühne als symbolisch wahrnehmen: "Es ist nichts theatralisch, was nicht für die Augen symbolisch wäre." (Goethe) Seine Wahrnehmung sollte entsprechend nicht seine Einfühlung ermöglichen, sondern seine Reflexion herausfordern.[30]

---

28 Friedrich Schiller, *Werke und Briefe*, vol. 8 (Frankfurt am Main: Deutscher Klassiker Verlag, 1992), 1085-87 (coauthored by Goethe and Schiller).

29 Erika Fischer-Lichte, "Theatralität: Zur Frage nach Kleists Theaterkonzeption" in *Kleist Jahrbuch 2001* (Stuttgart: Verlag J. B. Metzler, 2001), 25-37. For a more complete discussion, see also Erika Fischer-Lichte, *Theater im Prozeß der Zivilisation* (Tübingen: Franke, 2000).

30 Fischer-Lichte, "Theatralität," 32.

The "harmonic whole" of the aestheticized body on the Classical stage is not to be understood as representing a functional body in the way that the naturalized, affective, and semiotic body would strive to (despite the procedures of rendering the body as sign and the subsequent audience translation of this sign).[31] Rather, it should elicit a reflective awareness that forgets bodily presence in favor of the symbolic mode in which it operates as a static element of a tableau (*Staffage*: figure in a landscape, ornamental detail, decoration). One can see, in this distinction, how confusion might arise around the use of the word "natural" to designate on the one hand, the sniffling, fidgeting and coughing body that Goethe's "Regeln für Schauspieler" (*Rules for Actors*) seeks to ban from the theater – on both sides of the curtain – and the "natural" as idealized general-form theorized in Schiller's "Über den Gebrauch des Chors," on the other. Further, as evinced in the short, fragmentary essay "Über epische und dramatische Dichtung," the corollary effort in Weimar Classicism to define the classical genres complicates the understanding of the use of the aestheticized body on stage.

In its formulation of the characteristic difference between epic and dramatic poetry, the essay "Über epische und dramatische Dichtung" contrasts the medium, so to speak, of the voice with that of the body of the dramatic player. The voice of the rhapsodist or epic poet, the piece argues, should be heard as if from behind a curtain. It calls upon it's hearer to follow the evoked images through the use of the imaginative faculty over a broad and freely defined terrain.

> [M]an wird ihm (dem Rhapsodist) überall folgen, denn er hat es nur mit der Einbildungskraft zu tun, die sich ihre Bilder selbst hervorbringt.[32]

> His audience follows him (the Rhapsodist) wherever he leads because he is only appealing to the imagination, which creates its own images …[33]

The disembodied voice of the epic poet is argued to abstract all personality and cause its audience "to believe itself to hear only the voice of the muse in general" ("nur die Stimme der Musen im allgemeinen zu hören glauben") (1087). The *darstellende* efforts of the mime, the actor, on the other hand, constricts the free movement of the imaginative faculty and

31 For a dictionary of semiotics of the body contemporary to Weimar Classicism see Johann Jakob Engel, *Ideen zu einer Mimik* (Berlin, 1786).

32 Schiller with Goethe, *Werke und Briefe*, vol. 8 (Frankfurt am Main: Deutscher Klassiker Verlag, 1992), 1087.

33 Johann Wolfgang von Goethe, *Goethe's Collected Works*, vol. 3, *Essays on Art and Literature*, ed. John Gearey, trans. Ellen von Nardroff and Ernest H. von Nardroff (New York: Suhrkamp Publishers, 1986), 194.

gives rise to a feeling of *Mitleid.* (Here we immediately see an unexpected crossover into the terrain of *bürgerliches Trauerspiel*). This effect is produced by the presence of the body on stage and causes the audience to forget itself.

> Der Mime dagegen ist gerade in dem entgegengesetzten Fall; er stellt sich als ein bestimmtes Individuum dar, er will ... daß man die Leiden seiner Seele und seines Körpers mitfühle.[34]

> With the actor it is just the opposite. He represents a specific individual and wants us to concentrate exclusively on him and his immediate surroundings. His goal is to make us empathize with his mental anguish and his physical suffering, share his difficulties and forget ourselves.[35]

In this essay, Schiller and Goethe seem to be preoccupied with the recitation of poetry and the source of the voice that delivers the lines. Like a written text, the rhapsodist's presence should disappear before the imaging capacities of the imagination, whereas the actor's body announces itself. Despite the "distance" interposed between the symbolic body on stage and the audience's powers of reflection, in their distinction between genres Goethe and Schiller do not actually abandon some aspect of the affective immediacy of the theater. Dramatic art stills and enthralls its audience (termed "spectating listeners" in the essay) with the actor's body and the limits of the scene.

> Der zuschauende Hörer muß von Rechts wegen in einer steten sinnlichen Anstrengung bleiben, er darf sich nicht zum Nachdenken erheben, er muß leidenschaftlich folgen, seine Phantasie ist ganz zum Schweigen gebracht, man darf keine Ansprüche an sie machen, und selbst was erzählt wird, muß gleichsam darstellend vor die Augen gebracht werden.[36]

> It is an absolute necessity that the audience be constantly engaged and not be allowed to assume a position of detached contemplation. The actor wants them to be passionately involved and their imagination completely inactive; so he must not appeal to it, and even what is being narrated has to be made visual.[37]

According to Goethe and Schiller, the dramatic form manipulates the imaginative faculty in a manner directly opposed to that of the epic. The fact of scenic presentation immediately affects the conditions of poetic production and limits the capacity of the imagination for the free image-evocation that is enabled by recitation. In some sense, the audience for a

---

34 Schiller with Goethe, *Werke*, 1087

35 Goethe, *Goethe's Works*, 194.

36 Schiller with Goethe, *Werke*, 1087.

37 Goethe, *Works*, 194.

dramatic production is captive, and, as observed above, Schiller later reasoned that the insertion of the chorus between action and spectator could possibly mitigate against this loss of liberty. As we have seen with our brief excursus through the opening monologue of *Iphigenie auf Tauris*, these rules can have powerful consequences both for the promise of the dramatic plot and the scope of the social consequences of its performance. Not only that they insinuate a difference into the body on stage, a differencing within the self-same that opens to question the ambiguous relation, to speak once more with Kant, between the moral agent and the human subject, but precisely from the site of sacrifice and at the grounds of cultural alterity.

Kleist's Epic Poetics of the Stage

Though comprised predominantly of descriptive speech, of epic *Schilderung*, the stage for which *Penthesilea, Ein Trauerspiel* (1808) is written does not accommodate the stable and stately solemnity of the tragic player; words do not issue from characters, who, standing in one position, must somehow embody two.[38] Where Antigone must stand, accused, at once sister and subject, where Goethe's *Iphigenie auf Tauris* stands her ground for historical transformation, Penthesilea, as alien sovereign, may not stand still. Her speeches emerge within a nexus of reconstellating centers of power, so that if, like the traditional figure of tragedy, her position is always double, it is also ever differently double. Kleist's *Penthesilea* thus also shifts the space of the tragic stage, even further destabilizing the terms in which tragic representation can house the problems that haunt human action. A migratory faultline runs the length of the stage, which, as we shall see, also conditions the extent to which the figure Penthesilea has a claim or stake in the "human."

* * *

38 See also Vernant and Naquet, "Tensions and Ambiguities in Greek Tragedy" for a discussion of how doubleness might be at work in Ancient Greek tragedy as well. "All that the hero feels, says and does springs from his character, his *ethos*, which the poets analyze just as subtly and interpret just as positively as might, for example, the orators or a historian such as Thucydides. But at the same time these feelings, pronouncements, and actions also appear as the expression of a religious power, a *daimon* operating through them ... Thus every moment in the life of the hero unfolds as if on two levels. Each would, by itself, adequately account for the peripeteia of the drama, but the purpose of the tragedy is precisely to present them as inseparable ... For there to be tragedy it must be possible for the text simultaneously to imply two things: It is his character, in man, that one calls *daimon* and, conversely, what one calls character, in man, is in reality a *daimon*." (*Myth and Tragedy in Ancient Greece,* 37).

A contemporary critic of Kleist's, Karl August Böttiger writing for *Der Freimüthige* likened *Penthesilea* to the *Spektakelstücke* of the day, only worse. "The spectacle in this tragic drama is so mad that it couldn't be staged anywhere."[39] For evidence, Böttiger evokes the armies of the Greeks and Amazons ("girls and mothers – one can't call them women"), hounds and elephants, and finally Penthesilea's circus-size madness overloading the stage.[40] It is not only the unconventional personnel the critic deplores but the scale of Kleist's tragedy. His contention surprises, because the critic speaks here of a drama composed primarily of speech. These Kleistian words are too big. Indeed, the text of *Penthesilea* – never performed in Kleist's time and first attempted in 1876, sixty-five years after his death – continues to inspire a discussion of the limits and possibilities of the theater.

As we have seen in the discussion of "Über epische und dramatische Dichtung," Goethe and Schiller's definitions foreground the different responsive potentials ascribed to the imaginative faculty when forgetful of, or attuned to, the compassionate body. While the epic poet, a voice disembodied, frees the movement of the imagination, the body of the actor on stage restricts it. Embodying a concrete presence, the actor gives rise rather to an immediate feeling of *Mitleid* and – in contrast to the voice of the rhapsodist which engages the imagination's ability to generate its own images – the suffering body on stage enthralls the audience and brings the *Phantasie* "to silence."

Kleist's tragedy *Penthesilea* confounds the distinction between the epic and dramatic modes as outlined by Goethe and Schiller. The extensive employment of teichoscopy (*Mauerschau*) causes the Kleistian stage to be peopled by reports. Messengers strain to catch a glimpse of the events off-stage and recount these events in a volley of constantly interrupted and revised utterances. Witnesses call the gathered figures on stage to survive the recitation of gruesome events, and precisely the spectacle of the message conveyed and received fills and reorganizes the dimensions of the stage. Rather than emphasizing the limit of the stage, *Penthesilea* marks and springs this limit.[41] The body on the Kleistian stage already becomes a

---

39 *Der Freimüthige*, 5.2.1808. Böttiger's article is cited in the notes to Kleist, *Sämtliche Werke und Briefe*, vol. 2, 696. The piece is also to be found in Kleist's *Lebensspuren*, Nr. 225a.

40 Ibid.

41 In a collaborative comparative reading of *Penthesilea* and *Käthchen von Heilbronn*, Cullens and von Mücke argue that Kleist's use of the *Mauerschau* technique not only imitates but exceeds ancient convention. "Though the messenger report and the description of events taking place concurrently off-stage belong to the repertoire of the traditional tragedy, in the case of *Penthesilea* they are not employed so much to fill in gaps of information or to ac-

thing seen in the imagination *even* as it stands as the object of a sympathetic gaze. Precisely that engagement of the imagination attributed by Goethe and Schiller to the epic poet not only precedes the arrival of the actor but also accompanies the player's physical presence. Further, when the actor arrives, in this case Penthesilea, the report and her presence need not necessarily co-exist harmoniously. Rather, the two modes, the seen and the said, cross Kleist's stage in disjunction: at war.

Odysseus. ... und sie errinnert,
Daß sie mir noch die Antwort schuldig sei.
Drauf mit der Wangen Rot, wars Wut, wars Scham,
Die Rüstung wieder bis zum Gurt sich färbend,
Verwirrt und stolz und wild zugleich: sie sei
Penthesilea, kehrt sie zu mir,
Der Amazonen Königin, und werde
Aus Köchern mir die Antwort übersenden! (1.95-102)

Odysseus
... reminds her timidly
That she still owes an answer to my words.
Whether from rage or shame, another blush
Staining her harness crimson to the waist,
She turns to me, confusion, wildness, pride
Commingling in her face, and speaks: I am
Penthesilea, Queen of the Amazons,
And you shall have my arrows for reply! (8)

Penthesilea is first *heard* through indirect discourse and *appears* first in description. Bedecked with snake's heads and winding serpent-like out of the mountains, she rises up in Odysseus' speech and speaks indirectly through a gnarl of syntax that contains the dialogue of the stage within the recitation of the epic. Is it that she says she is Penthesilea, of the Amazon's Queen, or does Penthesilea, the Amazon's queen, turn to Odysseus? Where does the genetival phrase in apposition adhere: to the speech of Penthesilea as conveyed by Odysseus or to that part of the speech into which Odysseus intrudes with his narrative "sie kehrt"? In her first appearance, Penthesilea is already split in Odysseus' locution.

---

commodate what would violate the decorum of classical tragedy, but rather they disrupt the coherence of the scenic representation and call for the permanent revisions of what seems to have been established. In fact, they tend to destabilize the boundaries of the scene . . ." Chris Cullens and Dorothea von Mücke, "Love in Kleist's *Penthesilea* and *Käthchen von Heilbronn*," in *Deutsche Vierteljahrsschrift für Literaturwissenschaft und Geistesgeschichte* 63. no. 3 (1989): 463. See also Volker Klotz, "Aug um Zunge – Zunge um Aug, Kleist's extremes Theater," in *Kleist Jahrbuch* (1985): 128-42.

In the lines cited above, an elision is marked by a grammatical trace invisible to the audience. As in Samuel Beckett's stage direction at the beginning of *Ghost Trio: A Play for Television*, "Door ... Imperceptibly ajar,"[42] Kleist's tragic play calls for invisible presences on the stage and one aspect of it is secured only for readers. "Verwirrt und stolz und wild zugleich," the colon alone serves for Penthesilea's *sagen*, and serving in the place of the verb, it also functions as the sign of an equivalence: the copula or verb "to be." Odysseus' description attaches itself to Penthesilea's statement and a shadow of the imperative note in "*sie sei*" remains – calls Penthesilea to presence in an answer for which she is already guilty (*schuldig* – owes an answer).[43]

In fragmented and fierce descriptions, Odysseus tries to catch up with Penthesilea. One thinks of Lessing's remark in *Laokoon* that poetry allows the reader to hold mutually negating images in mind simultaneously. In Odysseus' opening monologue, her gender elided, Penthesilea is brought forth in the vein of the phenomenal and conveyed through epic simile. It's called Penthesilea, "Like hurricane wind torn from a cloud" ("Wie Sturmwind ein zerrissenes Gewölk") (Reese trans., 1.35). And alternately, as Odysseus states, "Here, this flat hand, I assure you,/is more expressive than her face" ("Hier diese flache Hand, versichr' ich dich,/Ist ausdrucksvoller als ihr Angesicht") (Reese trans., 1.66-67). Kleist's play introduces a figure at least temporarily unreadable and subject – open – to conjecture. Her body, her face is known from the start to reveal no expression. The drama immediately builds a flat plane, a wall or impasse, between the seer and the seen. The first thing the audience gets is Odysseus' hand across their eyes, as if the rhapsodist transposed himself between the actor and made the *Zuschauer* a *listener*. But even Odysseus' language cannot register the *Penthesilea* effect. Despite the exploitation of those capacities Lessing attributes to poetry, the problem of naming Penthesilea remains.

For Odysseus, himself the answerer of riddles (*Niemand*), Penthesilea presents the "nichts Drittes" between force and resistance (1.126). Her troops are observed as an effect the principle of which remains undivined. Through the confused attempt to describe this untenable "third" a kind of epic metaphorics of the stage arises that transforms the epic simile into a contiguous event – a dramatic action.

Ein Ätolier. Doch hinter ihm –
Der Hauptmann. Was?
Der Myrmidonier. An des Berges Saum –

---

42 Samuel Beckett, *Ends and Odds* (London: Faber & Faber, 1977).

43 This usage also recalls the Biblical imperative: "Es sei. Licht" (Let there be light) – as if offering to conjure her.

Der Ätolier. Staub –
Der Myrmidonier. Staub aufqualmend, wie Gewitterwolken:
Und, wie der Blitz vorzuckt –
Der Ätolier. Ihr ewgen Götter!
Der Myrmidonier. Penthesilea.
Der Hauptmann. Wer?
Der Ätolier. Die Königin! – (3.386-390)

An Etolian
Behind him, though –
Captain
What?
Myrmidon
By the moutain's edge –
Etolian
Dust –
Myrmidon
A smoke-like dust, dark, like a storm cloud:
And darting forth, like lightening –
Etolian
Deathless gods!
Myrmidon
Penthesilea.
Captain
Who?
Etolian
The Queen herself! – (19)

The reports delivered on Kleist's stage are subject to interjection, the interruption of astonishment, and to queries that break down into a rhythmic volley of answer and response among the figures on stage. Language is caught up in the specular, in a polyphony where answer and address suffer delay and run off, lines askew; in which "dust" and "Deathless gods!" serve to name as well as proper names and roles: "Penthesilea", "Königin." Here again, Kleist produces a reflexive and complex merger of the epic and dramatic modes as put forth in "Über epische und dramatische Dichtung." Goethe and Schiller differentiate the two modes with respect to the temporal status of the action:

> [I]hr großer wesentlicher Unterschied beruht aber darin, daß der Epiker die Begebenheit als *vollkommen vergangen* vorträgt, und der Dramatiker sie als *vollkommen gegenwärtig* darstellt.[44]

> The fundamental difference between them is that the epic writer narrates an event as having happened in the past, while the dramatist represents an event as happening in the present.[45]

---

44 Schiller with Goethe, *Werke und Briefe*, 1085-87.

In the above-cited excerpts, the actions at issue are neither past nor properly present; rather, they cast their influence over the stage from some point beyond and produce a strange poetry of testimony and interjection. Unlike Goethe's *Iphigenie auf Tauris*, who mediates between the particular and general as exemplary instance, the barely glimpsed and ajar presences on Kleist's stage neither take place in monologue nor in eloquent acts of self-determination. Rather, they emerge in exclamations of astonishment, in scenes of interrupted and startled witness, and from producers of effects (*Staub aufqualmend)*. The concretized epic of Kleist's stage seems less to harmonize the ideal with the real, than to shake the two apart, leaving trails and resonances between the *Staffage* of the human body on stage and its lyric enunciation in words. The events are *present* and *unseen* and then *present, seen* and unrecognizable. Within this paradox rests the concretized figurative: "Staub" refers directly, "Gewitterwolk" through likeness describes, "Penthesilea" names, but each designation becomes address, word, and thing within the performance of the play.

Hundekomödie: Dog Theater

> Komödienzettel.
> Heute zum ersten Mal mit Vergunst: die Penthesilea,
> Hundekomödie; Acteure: Helden und Köter und Fraun.[46]
> – Heinrich von Kleist, Phöbus Fragmente

Böttiger does not go far enough in noticing that armies encumber Kleist's stage: they actually take possession of it. At the end of Scene 9, the Priestesses and Rose-Maidens flee the scene as Amazon soldiers approach to ward off Achilles, who is also perilously near. In Scene 17, Diomedes and

45 Goethe, *Goethe's Works*, 192.

46 In the April/May edition of the *Phöbus*, Kleist published a series of epigrams, several on the subject of *Penthesilea* and the piece's negative critical reception. The epigraph above is the second of these. As I hope my argument will show, this description is more than self-persiflage, beating his critic to the punch. It's also a straightforward description, for the prime category under seige in Kleist's revisititation of the dramas of Greek antiquity is the "human." There are multiple versions of the sub- and superhuman which comprise the metaphorics of his verse, that is, dogs, heroes and women. If at the beginning of the 22nd Scene, a confusion arises between the plural "die" to indicate "the dogs" and "die" to indicate the "Die Königin," by the 23rd scene Penthesilea has become "Sie, die fortan kein Name nennt – " (23.2607). (She who no name any longer names…) As the High Priestess says: "Laß sie/Gebirge decken, unzugängliche,/Und den Gedanken deiner Tat dazu! War ich's, du – Mensch nicht mehr, wie nenn' ich dich?" (24.2728-2731) On the other hand, the Amazons are "human" and they are fighting for "fatherland." Kleist's play concerns "the human" and the battles taking place across the word, the fragile space of that stage. "Ach! Wie gebrechlich ist der Mensch, ihr Götter!" (24.3037)

Odysseus try to persuade Achilles to abandon the stage as another band of Amazon soldiers draws on, and in Scene 18, Amazon troops reclaim both the stage and its heroine, Penthesilea. In this way, the stage becomes the scene of reconstellating spheres of influence that determine and reconstrue the possibility of speech. The *place* which holds a particular dialogue dissolves at the approach of new forces. Diomedes: "Vom Platz hier fort, Doloperheld! Vom Platze!" ("Dolopian hero, leave this place! Away!") and Odysseus: "Fort! Rasender!/Hier ist der Ort nicht mehr, zu trotzen" ("Leave!/Defy them somewhere else, you maniac! [literally "Here is the place no longer,"]) (17.2274 and 18.2295-6). Single point perspective, the Olympian view or vantage of the *Feldherr*, surveying from a prominence and constructing a hierarchical, homogenous space, is missing.[47] In this the compelling *and* ideal body of Goethe and Schiller's description is sprung into complexity. The body on stage takes on a sheer poetic proximity to animals, words and things. Undermining the classical generic divisions of Weimar, Kleist's approach to theater fractures vision and introduces a heterogeneous, contested space subject to de- and reterritorializations.[48] There is no permanence of place within the action of *Penthesilea* but rather a series of occupations (*Besetzungen*) that bring fleeting encampments of gesture and usage to the stage.

In crucial Scene 15, "the love scene," the approaching Amazon company forces Achilles' courtly language to give up the lie. They impel his metaphors of surrender to reveal themselves as issuing from the condition of Penthesilea's captivity. Similarly, Penthesilea implores Achilles to understand that there are words that can only be delivered and received in particular places.

Penthesilea. O Neridensohn!
Du willst mir nicht nach Themiscrya folgen?
Du willst mir nicht zu jenem Tempel folgen,
Der aus den fernen Eichenwipfeln ragt?
Komm her, ich sagte dir noch alles nicht –
Achilles. (*nun völlig gerüstet, tritt vor sie und reicht ihr die Hand*).
Nach Phtia, Kön'gin.
Penthesilea. O! - Nach Themiscrya!
O! Freund! Nach Themiscrya, sag ich dir,
Wo Dianas Tempel aus den Eichen ragt!
Und wenn der Sel'gen Sitz in Phtia wäre,

47 Cullens and von Mücke, "Love in Kleist's *Penthesilea* and *Käthchen von Heilbronn*," 464.

48 See Wolf Kittler, *Geburt des Partisanen aus dem Geist der Poesie* (Freiburg im Breisgau: Rombach Verlag, 1987) for a fascinating discussion of partisan tactics of war and Kleist's poetics.

doch, doch, o Freund! nach Themiscrya noch,
Wo Dianas Tempel aus den Wipfeln ragt!
Achilles. (*indem er sie aufhebt*).
So mußt du mir vergeben, Teuerste;
Ich bau dir solchen Tempel bei mir auf. (17.2280-2292)

Penthesilea
Son of the Nereid!
You will not follow me to Themiscrya?
You will not follow me to that fair temple
That rises tall among the distant oaks?
Come here, I haven't told you everything –
Achilles
My Queen – to Phthia.
Penthesilea
Oh! – To Themsicrya!
Oh! Friend! I tell you, it's to Themsicrya
Where Diana's temple looms above the oaks!
And if in Phthia the Blessed had their dwelling,
Still, still, oh friend! it's still to Themiscrya!
Where Diana's temple looms above the oaks!
Achilles
(lifting her up)
You must forgive me, then, my precious one.
I'll build you another temple just like yours. (106-107)

Between Penthesilea's "jenem" and Achilles' "solchen," the tension lies. The repetition in these verses emphasizes the impossibility of transplanting the temple or translating what it does to words. The significance of the temple can only be intimated by the repetition of its name, its formulaic attributes, the injunction to go there. The exchange of vows between Penthesilea and Achilles, precariously held in a fleeting détente, occurs at the center of a losing and giving of ground and cannot escape the exigencies of place that both prepare and threaten this exchange. Thus, Achilles "tears" her away as she was also "ripped" from the throne to engage in the Amazonian war-hunt.[49] In the war hunt there are no treaties. Kleist fashions a zone wherein all translations are forced, in that warring principles of war variously occupy and flee his stage.

Much has been written of the Amazonian mode of war with reference to Odysseus' opening monologues.[50] Odysseus operates as the tragedy's

---

49 *Penthesilea. – Lange weint ich ... Bis mich zu letzt der wiederholte Ruf*
Des Volks ... Gewaltsam auf den Thron riß (15.2150-57).

50 See Wolf Kittler, *Die Geburt des Partisanen aus dem Geist der Poesie*, 218-324. Also Gilles Deleuze and Félix Guattari, *A Thousand Plateaus*, trans. Brian Massumi (Minneapolis: University of Minnesota Press, 1987), 354-56. See also Manfred Schneider, "Die Welt im Aus-

first informant concerning the Amazons and their actions, but he is an informant with limited knowledge. As such, his testimonies frame subsequent actions in a mood of astonishment and disbelief. Part of the ambiguity of the Amazons rests in the problem that it is impossible to discern what they want. Agamemnon reasons, speaking through Antilochus, that if the Amazon battle is abandoned and Penthesilea pursues Achilles to Troy, then in the sight of Agamemnon's helmsmanship she will be decided.

Antilochus. Verfolgt sie euch, so wird er, der Atride,
Dann an des Heeres Spitze selber sehn,
Wozu sich diese rätselhafte Sphinx
Im Angesicht von Troja wird entscheiden. (1.205-208)

Antilochus
Should she pursue you, he, the son of Atreus,
Will, at the army's head, find out himself
What purpose guides this enigmatic Sphinx
Who comes to battle by the gates of Troy. (11)

For the Greeks, "the face of Troy" provides the locus of determinacy and legibility. In Troy, Penthesilea will be *brought* to comprehension; or more properly, to combat. This is not the divination of the riddle, but its obsolescence. The mystery extends beyond Penthesilea, since she has also managed to riddle Greek speech. For this reason not even repetition can secure the meaning of a word or name as Penthesilea had tried with the name "Themiscrya." In one unusual point of commonality in their usage, the phrase "word for word" passes between the Greeks and Amazons alike; as when Antilochus replies to Odysseus' first long speech characterizing Penthesilea (discussed extensively above): "So, word for word, your messenger reported;/But no one in the entire Grecian camp,/Could comprehend it" ("So, Wort für Wort, der Bote, den du sandtest;/Doch keiner in dem ganzen Griechenlager,/Der ihn begriff") (1.103-5). Like Penthesilea repeating "Themiscrya" to Achilles, the Greeks are left repeating messages word for word without being able to grasp them – or have them convey. By bringing Penthesilea to resistance or complicity, the strategizing Greeks hope to retrieve comprehensibility to their own side.

The problem of comprehensibility "on one's own side" must teach *Penthesilea*'s reader-viewer to read-look beyond Odysseus' model of force

---

nahmezustand", 115-16. Schneider connects the logic of the Amazon state to a "dark, biopolitical frenzy" arguing: "Es ist also nicht aktualisierter Mythos, sondern die biopolitische Staatsraison des 18. Jahrhunderts, die den Grund des Amazonenkriegs bildet." Not actualized myth, but biopolitical state's reason founds the Amazon war ethic. The question still remains, why they're dressed up as "Amazons" in order to perform this function.

and its resistance. This formula should be analogically transposed onto that of the gender dyad no more than the the difference between the Amazons and the Greeks should be construed in a leveling formal equivalence (i.e., that they are different in the same way, to the same degree). Their ignorance is not mutual. The Amazons are not beyond distinguishing between the Greek campaigners. When Asteria attests that she came only as a spectator, knowing herself unnecessary where victory was already assured, she also describes her disappointment.

Asteria. Neugierde treibt mich doch, die Schar zu sehen,
Die man mir als des Sieges Beute rühmt;
Und eine Handvoll Knechte, bleich und zitternd,
Erblickt mein Auge, der Argiver Auswurf,
Auf Schildern, die sie fliehend weggeworfen,
Von deinem Kriegstroß schwärmend aufgelesen.
Vor Trojas stolzen Mauern steht das ganze
Hellenheer, steht Agamemmnon noch,
Stehn Menelaus, Ajax, Palamed;
Ulysses, Diomedes, Antilochus ... (5.767-75)

Asteria
Curiosity,
Though, prods me to examine what we've won,
The band of youths whose praises I've been hearing.
And there I find a sad handful of slaves,
Pale, shivering, the Argives' dregs,
Picked up like gleanings by your baggage train
And carried off on shields they'd thrown away.
Outside the lofty walls of Troy there stands
The whole Hellenic army: Agamemmnon,
And Menelaos, and Ajax, Palamede;
Odysseus, Diomede, Antilochus ... (35)

Asteria can name the Greek heroes in litany and, apparently, identify them as well. She is already Greek-literate before she arrives. I wish to emphasize this, for while the Amazons are wildly strange to the Greeks, the Amazonian society is not a pre-Trojan war society but rather one that has incorporated the fame of the venging Greeks.[51] In the encyclopedic love scene between Achilles and Penthesilea, during which accounts of identity and origin are exchanged, it is in fact Penthesilea who recites Achilles'

---

51 See Carol Jacobs, *Uncontainable Romanticism*, 85-114. The introduction to her argument points both to Penthesilea as reader of the *Iliad* and Kleist's *Penthesilea* as the text that unravels the classical source by killing its hero. Not broken up into Acts and Scenes, the play is comprised of twenty-four consecutive scenes, suggesting an allusion to the number of Books of Homer's *Iliad*.

story as well as her own.[52] Not only did her mother name him, but the valleys themselves resound with the fame of the Trojan war.

Penthesilea. Mein ewiger Gedanke, wenn ich wachte,
Mein ewger Traum warst du! Die ganze Welt
Lag wie ein ausgespanntes Musternetz
Vor mir; in jeder Masche, weit und groß,
War deiner Taten eine eingeschürzt
Und in mein Herz, wie Seide weiß und rein,
Mit Flammenfarben jede brannt ich ein. (15.2187-93)

Penthesilea
My one unending thought when I was waking,
My endless dream, was you! The entire world
Lay stretched before me like a patterned web
With wide and ample meshes, and each one
Had one of your deeds woven into it,
And into my heart, white and pure as silk,
I branded each of them with flaming colors. (102)

Penthesilea has not only read the *Iliad* but has already incorporated the fabled Achilles. Ever the huntress, she intends to mark and adorn herself with another's fame: a fame widely appreciated.[53] In one sense, the Amazons are connoisseurs in the Greek marketplace. For this reason, the Amazon-Greek difference cannot be construed as a pure difference in terms of a formal equality; they are not, in other words, different from one another in the same way. There is a disequilibrium at the core of their encounter, the pivot point of which is cultural literacy. Though the Amazon mode of the hunt is predicated on a principle of randomness, their appraisal of its gains appears not to be random. Penthesilea is aware of the woman-customs of the Greeks and knows herself strange to them (15.1889-97). Achilles moves within the medium of his ignorance, his fascination with the sudden descent of Penthesilea "as if descended from the clouds" ("wie aus den Wolken nieder"), and his somewhat graceless wish to know: "Be more specific" ("Sei deutlicher"), he demands as Penthesilea works out remote origins (15.1912). Penthesilea cannot claim the same ignorance of Achilles.

---

52 In a later section I will discuss the fact that Achilles *has* heard of the legend of the Amazons, for he does say at one point, "It's true then." The encounter with an Amazon is an encounter with a legend come to life.

53 *Penthesilea. Auf allen Märkten, hohe Lieder schallen,*
Die des Hero'nkriegs Taten feierten:
Vom Paris-Apfel, dem Helenenraub ... (15.2119-2121)

Some efforts have been made to diagnose Penthesilea in the secondary literature.[54] These readings, however, must first transpose the action of the tragic play into narrative form. Such narrativization, however, is forged from an assemblage of speeches that cannot *grasp* each other on stage. The flights and lapses of consciousness that characterize Penthesilea's utterances mirror the battle for the stage and its legibility – and this battle takes place on all sides of the action. A thematic of *vernehmen* and *schildern* runs through the dialogue of *Penthesilea*. These actions of hearing and listening take place in the rifts that open in and through resistance to comprehension, in the sense both of the ability to understand and that of being included, contained.

References to the Medusa proliferate throughout the play as different speeches and actions freeze their listeners. Meroe calls herself the *afrikanische Gorgone* as she prepares to tell the horrifying story of Penthesilea's deed and closes by calling her audience to wake from the graven immobility caused by the tale.

Meroe. Die Afrikanische Gorgone bin ich,
Und wie ihr steht, zu Steinen starr ich euch.
. . . .

54 See Joachim Pfeiffer, "Kleists 'Penthesilea' Eine Deutung unter den Aspekten von narzißtischer und ödipaler Problematik" in *Kontroversen alte und neue: Akten des III. Internationalen Germanistischen Kongresses*, ed. Albrecht Schöne (Göttingen 1985), 196: "In Kleists Drama finden wir einen Schauplatz, auf dem sich die Protagonisten – Penthesilea and Achill – weit vom Realitätsprinzip entfernen…." See also, Falk Horst, "Kleists Penthesilea oder die Unfähigkeit, aus Liebe zu kämpfen", in *Germanisch-Romanische Monatsschrift* 36, no. 2 (1986): 150-68, which treats of contradictions between Amazon prescription and "Gefühlsbindung u. Selbstbestimmung." For readers of *Penthesilea,* the problem of what to do with these Amazons has been crucial. Readings that assume the society of Amazons a travesty have read the tragedy as complete at the onset, i.e., Penthesilea's "downfall" as proceeding cleanly and singly out of her participation in an unnatural order. For instance; Albert Sieck's view: "Der tötende erotische Verschlingungstrieb Penthesileas … ist das, was sich aus ihrem Amazonentum entwickelt" (cited in Angress, "Kleist's Nation of Amazons," 108). Angress points out that these arguments overlook the pivot point of identification between Penthesilea and Achilles: corpse desecration. The act and sign of her "downfall" draws her into community with the Greek hero in transgression of the Amazon law, therefore the tragedy little seems the putting on trial of the latter. See also Walter Müller-Seidel, *Versehen und Erkennen: Eine Studie über Heinrich von Kleist* (Cologne: Bohlau, 1961), in which the opinion is expressed that the catastrophe derives from the "Scheingesetz" of the Amazons. Vestiges of this view linger in some contemporary interpretations that read the symptoms of Penthesilea's fractured subjectivity on the body that marks her as an Amazon. Helga Gallas' reading with Lacan's *Four Discourses* names the lost breast as the "auffälligste Symptom" of "ein gespaltenes ... haltloses Subjekt" (Helga Gallas, "Kleists *Penthesilea* und Lakans vier Diskurse," in *Kontroversen, alte und neue. Akten des VII. Kongresses der Internationalen Vereinigung der germanistischen Sprach- und Literaturwissenschaft*, ed. Albrecht Schöne [Tübingen 1986], 6: 203-212). This argument, however, founders on overdetermination – if all subjects are split then why does the Amazon breast serve as the symptom?

(*Pause voll Entsetzen*)
Vernahmt ihr mich, ihr Fraun, wohlan, so redet,
und gebt ein Zeichen eueres Lebens mir. (23.2603-4 and 23.2675-76)

Meroe
I am the Gorgon come of Africa,
And as you stand, my stare turns you to stone.
. . . .
If you have heard me, women, speak to me,
Give me a sign that you still live and breathe.

Meroe's mode of recitation opposes that suggested above by Goethe and Schiller. The speaker becomes not the veiled voice of the Muse but a menacing figure whose speech stares her audience to stone. The imaginative faculty does not range freely in her words but is driven to a grim constriction. Later, the High Priestess tells Penthesilea – whose body is gradually becoming language as the action of the play advances, "Du blickst die Ruhe meines Lebens tot." In this use of *blicken*, Kleist makes the verb "to glance or gaze" transitive so that Penthesilea has "glanced the repose of my life dead." Penthesilea herself laments, after her fatefully deluded revelation of her origins: "Ein steinern Bild hat meine Hand bekranzt" ("My hand garlanded a stone image"). The figure for elucidation on the Kleistian stage is Medusa. Scenes of explanation do not bring about reconciliation but lead to freezes or flights of consciousness, to the lightening shock of vision, or to the sudden transformation of the living into an uninterpretable bas-relief. Here I recall Penthesilea's immobility in the face of Odysseus' persistent questioning, his moment of ambassadorial welcome.

Gedankenvoll, auf einen Augenblick,
Sieht sie in unsre Schar, von Ausdruck leer,
Als ob in Stein gehau'n wir vor ihr stünden;
Hier diese flache Hand, versich'r ich dich,
Ist ausdrucksvoller als ihr Angesicht:
Bis jetzt ihr Aug auf den Peliden trifft ... (1.63-68)

For one long moment, with a pensive gaze
She stares into our ranks, void of expression,
As if we stood before her carved in stone;
This bare flat palm has more expressive features
Than were displayed upon that woman's face:
Until her glance meets that of Peleus' son: ... (7)

As the strange logic of the Penthesilea-Achilles hunt-courtship progresses, comprehensibility becomes increasingly at risk "on both sides." Odysseus cannot cause Achilles to attend – neither to listen nor to return to Troy.

Odysseus. (indem er die Arme verschränkt).
- Ich kanns nicht glauben.

Achilles. Er spricht von der Dardanerburg.
Odysseus. Was?
Achilles. Was?
Odysseus. Mich dünkt, du sagtest was.
Achilles. Ich?
Odysseus. Du!
Achilles. Ich sagte:
Er spricht von der Dardanerburg.
Odysseus. Nun ja!
Wie ein Beseßner fragt ich, ob der ganze
Helenenstreit, von der Dardanerburg,
Gleich einem Morgentraum, vergessen sei?
Achilles. (in dem er näher tritt).
Wenn die Dardanerburg, Laertiade,
Versänke, du verstehst, so daß ein See,
Ein bläulicher, an ihre Stelle träte;
Wenn graue Fischer, bei dem Schein des Monds,
Den Kahn an ihre Wetterhähne knüpften;
Wenn im Palast des Priamus ein Hecht
Regiert', ein Ottern- oder Ratzenpaar
Im Bette sich der Helena umarmten:
So wärs für mich gerad so viel, als jetzt. (21.2512-2526)

Odysseus
(crossing his arms)
I can't believe it.
Achilles
He talks about the walls of Troy.
Odysseus
What?
Achilles
What?
Odysseus
I thought you said something.
Achilles
I?
Odysseus
You!
Achilles
I said:
He talks about the walls of Troy.
Odysseus
Well, yes!
I asked him, like a man possessed, if Helen
And our great fight before the walls of Troy
Have been forgotten, like a morning dream?
Achilles
(stepping up closer to him)

> Son of Laertes, if the walls of Troy
> Should sink, you understand, so that a lake,
> A bluish one, replaced the battlements;
> And if at night gray fishermen attached
> Their boat by moonlight to the weathercocks;
> And if a pike were lord in Priam's palace,
> And if in Helen's bed a pair of otters,
> Or, say, a pair of water rats, embraced:
> It would mean just the same to me as now. (121)

A broken circuit of answer and address characterizes the dialogue that leads to Achilles' absurd repetitions. Odysseus' accusation that Achilles has forgotten the Greek campaign meets its consummation in Achilles' brightly sarcastic speech. Indeed, like a dream just before morning, Achilles speaks the Greek history out of existence and casts his indifference in mock-epic vein. Not only does Achilles drown the scene of the great battle, but he evacuates the names of sense. "Dardanerburg" is flattened out; it no longer serves as a prominence. Achilles performs here the alienation of context that characterizes Odysseus', admittedly more fiery, opening evocation of the Amazons.

Not only are names deflated, shorn of sense, or rendered obsolete in the play, but in many ways the violent actions described on the stage of *Penthesilea* comprise a battle for names. Out of the sea that Achilles makes of the Trojan battlefield, arises a fight for the possession of the name "Penthesilea." As Achilles gradually comes to be the last Greek visible on the stage – even if a corpse – all assembled compete for the territory of "Penthesilea."

From the outset, the Greek reporter announces: "Penthesilea, hieß es" (loosely: "Penthesilea, it goes" or "Penthesilea, it was said") to describe the battle. A similar elision of gender occurs when the Amazon speaker, speaking her name for the last time, shifts back into the neutral *es* of "das Wort." Likened to animals throughout by the Greeks, she finally loses her name as the Amazons take on the Greek usage and themselves see her as "den grimmigen Hunden beigesellt." Becoming her deed as mediated through Meroe's speech, she approaches: "Die Amazone. Hier kommt es, bleich, wie eine Leiche, schon/Das Wort des Greuelrätsels uns heran" ("The Amazons: Here it comes, pale, like a corpse/The answer [word] to the gruesome riddle approaches") (Reese translation, 24.2599-600). Where previously "Penthesilea" had been the war cry of the Amazons, "Und ihre Losung ist: Penthesilea!" ("And their battle cry is: Penthesilea!") they must now renounce her name (16.2264). Interesting to note, the scene preceding the war cry "Penthesilea" is the fifteenth scene in which Penthesilea offers her name to Achilles, which he repeats and then appropriates in a moment of exceedingly black humor:

Penthesilea. Ich bin die Königin der Amazonen,
Er nennt sich marserzeugt, mein Völkerstamm,
Otrere war die große Mutter mir,
Und mich begrüßt das Volk: Penthesilea.
Achilles. Penthesilea.
Penthesilea. Ja, so sagt ich dir.
Achilles. Mein Schwan singt noch im Tod: Penthesilea. (15.1824-30)

Penthesilea
Then know I am the Queen of the Amazons;
Of Mars begotten is my ancient tribe,
The famed Otrerë was my noble mother,
Myself the people call: Penthesilea.
Achilles
Penthesilea.
Penthesilea
Yes, so I did say.
Achilles
My swan in death shall sing: Penthesilea. (89)

As if indeed this name has the empty ring of an unknown word, he repeats it, fully enticed by what Penthesilea later understands is the "Musik der Rede." That the Amazons, after this exchange, will finally override Penthesilea's will and save her seems partly motivated by the need to reclaim her from Achilles' empty repetition of her name, which verges on a faulty translation. At the idyllic center of these contending similes Achilles seems to manage to bring the central name around which all figures on stage place themselves into pure sound.

The stage, providing no stable point of reference, passes over from the domain of one metaphor to another: the Greeks describing the Amazons, the Amazons describing the Greeks. As such, each account is already filtered by its contact with and resistance against its opponent. Achilles, the rising sun of Greek description, becomes a slender-necked doe in Amazon territory and Penthesilea's frantic quest before the steep cliff reveals for the Greeks "ein Wunsch, der keine Flügel hat" (*a wish, which has no wings*). Nonetheless, some wordcurrents surge through the various usages of Kleist's stage. The impossibility of "comprehensibility" opens onto a figure of rupture and flight. The Greeks "vereint" (united) against Achilles seek to direct him back to where his business lies. They propose, through the arts of speech, to use "Vernunft keilförmig, mit Gelassenheit" (*Reason, like a wedge, calmly*) (Reese translation, 1.230) to convince him of his error and separate him from his mistaken intentions.

Meanwhile, the figure of Penthesilea ranges wildly before the rocks, seeking "jeden sanftern Riß" (*every softer fissure*) that might break the impasse and lead her to her quarry. The High Priestess also uses the operative terms of the rent or tear to condemn Penthesilea to her decisions:

> Die Oberpriesterin. Frei, in des Volkes Namen, sprech ich dich;
> Du kannst den Fuß jetzt wenden, wie du willst,
> Kannst ihn mit flatterndem Gewand ereilen,
> Der dich in Fesseln schlug, und ihm den Riß,
> Da, wo wir sie zersprengten, überreichen ... (19.2329-2333)

> The High Priestess
> Free, in our people's name, I now pronounce you,
> And you may wend your feet wherever you please,
> May run with fluttering garments after him
> Who clapped you in irons, and bring back to him
> The bonds we broke, for mending. (110)

The "flatterndes Gewand" in this passage harks back to another of Penthesilea's gloriously deluded monologues. She dreams herself in Themiscrya, preparing for the *Rosenfest*, and calls to her maidens: "Und all ihr flatternden Gewänder, schürzt euch,/Ihr goldenen Pokale, füllt euch an" (14.1653-4). These wind-fluttered garments of the open field gathered up for celebration seem to be the trope of an Amazonian freedom. In Penthesilea's new freedom delivered through the Priestesses' words, however, the freedom of the "rent" chain must lead rather to collapse. As in scene 10, in Meroe's words: "Da fällt sie leblos,/Wie ein Gewand, in unsrer Hand zusammen." (*There she falls, liveless,/Like a gown, in our hands*) (10.1389-90).[55] As seen in the strange mix of the dramatic with the epic, actions always come within their filtering words, and words are born up in the stress of actions, which cannot exclusively possess them. Penthesilea as battle cry and swan song: the dire proximity of the promise and the slip of the tongue for which Kleist's play is famous. *Versprechen*, to promise, to speak oneself *over to* another may soon fall into the reflexive problem of an

---

55 In Penthesilea's final revelation scene, the ungraspable "word for word" of the Greek message returns in which Penthesilea argues, she was not so mad.

> *Penthesilea. ...Sieh her: als ich an deinem Halse hing,*
> *Hab ichs wahrhaftig Wort für Wort getan;*
> *Ich war nicht so verrückt, als es wohl schien.* (24. 2997-2999)

In her argument, Carol Jacobs insists upon a fundamental difference between this "word for word" and that of the Greeks. On the other hand, it is of note that just this phrase passes back and forth between encampments.

inadvertent slip, *sich versprechen*.[56] In the attempt to pass over, metaphor demands metamorphosis. Here, language either collapses or produces something unrecognizable leading to the commission of unnameable deeds. It is the unnameable deed, meanwhile, that lies at the root of the Penthesilea-Achilles identificatory collapse.[57]

Origin Stories and the Giving of Ground

Gérard Genette terms the denouement of Heinrich von Kleist's *Penthesilea, Ein Trauerspiel* (1808), "the triumph of phantasm."[58] In this he refers to Kleist's treatment of the classical antecedents on which the play draws:

> The pragmatic transformation is a bold one, since it does away with the hallowed tradition of Achilles' invulnerability and his subsequent feats until Paris' arrow, guided by Apollo, strikes him down. It amounts to a complete axiological inversion in relation to the data of the hypotext: it is no longer Achilles who experiences guilt and wretchedness after Penthesilea's death; the obverse occurs, and in the most atrocious manner. The victim becomes the executioner and the executioner the victim ... none, to my knowledge, assigns the final victory to Penthesilea and death to Achilles. The chosen variant is at all events the sole responsibility of the poet...[59]

Kleist's chosen variant is not a variant, but an invention. Though several different versions of her confrontation with Achilles were obtainable in Kleist's source in Hederich's dictionary of mythology,[60] Penthesilea was more prevalent on funerary urns than in poetry in the Classical Age and

---

56 In the final scene just as one might expect a moment of *agnorisis* parallel to that of Agave in Euripides' *Bacchae*, Penthesilea only says, "Du Ärmster aller Menschen, du vergibst mir!/Ich habe mich, bei Diana, bloß versprochen" (24.2985-86).

57 I rely here on Ruth Angress's careful comparison of the *Iliad* and *Penthesilea* and her demonstration that Penthesilea and Achilles become identified with each other as corpse desecrators. If anything, she learns it from him and Kleist's play is clear on this. Ruth Angress, "Kleist's Nation of Amazons," 101-107.

58 Girard Genette, *Palimpsests: Literature in the Second Degree* (Lincoln: University of Nebraska Press, 1997), 375-76.

59 Ibid., 376.

60 Benjamin Hederich, *Gründliches Mythologisches Lexikon* (Darmstadt: Wissenschaftliche Buchgesellschaft, 1996). Facsimile reprint of 1770 original. Genette may not have been aware of Hederich, generally assumed to have been one of Kleist's sources, as the entry in that dictionary does outline one variant wherein Penthesilea first slays Achilles who is then revived by Zeus at the pleading of Thetis. I am not aware of any variant in which Penthesilea and not Achilles becomes a corpse-desecrator. In this sense, Genette's primary point still holds. See Ruth Angress's discussion of Kleist's reference to the *Iliad*. "Kleist's Nation of Amazons" in *Beyond the Eternal Feminine: Critical Essays on Women and German Literature* (Stuttgart: Akademischer Verlag Hans-Dieter Heinz, 1982), 101-7.

was perhaps more familiar to Heinrich von Kleist from seventeenth and eighteenth century opera.[61] Further, what written mention of Penthesilea did acquire in the extant ancient Greek texts was to be found in the epic and not the dramatic tradition.[62] One is tempted to imagine that in some sense Kleist took his inspiration, as was often the case, from a precedent image rather than a precedent text.[63] On this occasion, though, Kleist may have relied on something more like a "mental image": the imagining of an "Amazon queen" and the possibilities conjured in such an enunciation or proposition. The one surviving element of his sources to which his *Penthesilea* does adhere is the report that there was a battle between Achilles and the Amazon Penthesilea that may have ended in the desecration of her corpse.[64] As Genette points out, the roles of victim and assailant are reversed and this reversal forms the crux of Kleist's *Trauerspiel*'s intertext.

The issue of how foundations are laid is repeated at many junctures within the drama's development and forms the pivotal theme in Scene 15, the "love scene" of verbal, non-agonistic exchange between Achilles and Penthesilea. Written within the context of Weimar Classicism, which defines itself in response to the cultural enterprise of "laying foundations" and generating a symbolic form that unifies the ideal with the actual, Kleist's *Penthesilea* can be argued to reflect on this process through its incorporation of a scene of exchange that unveils the origin of a social order and its foundational law.

Kleist's play incorporates a central scene in which a "Volk" expounds itself not so much as a play within a play, but as a play which choreo-

---

61 As the editors note in the Deutscher Klassiker Verlag edition of Kleist's plays: "Zu Kleists Zeit waren die Amazonen vor allem durch bildliche Darstellungen (u.a. auf einigen Metopen des Schatzhauses der Athener in Delphi um 500 v.Chr.; auf einer Metope des Hera-Tempels in Selinunt, 460-450 v. Chr., und auf mehreren rotfigurigen Vasen des 6. und 5. Jahrhunderts v. Chr.) gibt es gemalte Amazonenschlachten von Giulio Romano (1499-1546) in Mantua, von L. Cimbiaso (1527-1585) in Genua, von P. Schoubroeck (um 1570-1607) in Dresden, von Peter Paul Rubens (1577 bis 1640) in München, von P. Liberi (1614-1687) in Chambéry, von L. Giordano (1632-1705) in Neapel und in Wien. ... Außerdem hatten eine Reihe von Opern verschiedene Aspekte des Amazonen-Mythos zum Gegenstand ... " (691).

62 Robert Graves notes, "Penthesilea does not appear in the *Iliad*, but Achilles's outrage of her corpse is characteristically Homeric, and since she is mentioned in so many other Classical texts, a passage about her may well have been suppressed by Peisistratus's editors" (Robert Graves, *The Greek Myths*, vol. 2 [Baltimore: Penguin, 1959], 319).

63 Kleist claims an etching gave impetus to his comedy *Der Zerbrochene Krug*: "Ich nahm die Veranlassung dazu aus einem Kupferstich ... ." Heinrich von Kleist, *Sämtliche Werke und Briefe*, vol. 1, ed. Ilse-Marie Barth et al. [Frankfurt am Main: Deutscher Klassiker Verlag, 1987], 259).

64 Reclam's *Erläuterungen und Dokumente* series provides a good compilation of source texts for Kleist's *Penthesilea*, (*Heinrich von Kleist: "Penthesilea"* [Stuttgart: Reclam, 1992], 51-69).

graphs a contest for the stage. Penthesilea's recitation of the origins of the Amazonian "Frauenstaat" thus touches upon the active project of a theater to shed the modern garments that clothe the audience to expose the truly human in idealized form on stage. The irony, however, lies in part in casting Achilles as the one who receives the legend. In contradistinction to Goethe's Iphigenie, who recounts her own myth in monologue, Penthesilea's exposition of foundations takes place at the site of an exchange. It is within the fleeting idyllic caesura in this battle for ground that Penthesilea narrates the origin of the "Amazon state" in a scene also riven by the dramatic irony of Achilles' sham captivity. Achilles is the privileged recipient of her enunciation – a demand for an account of their origins had already been refused once when made in the first scene by Odysseus. As Antilochus had stated clearly in the opening scene of the play: "Und niemand kann, was sie uns will, ergründen." Achilles takes over the placeholder, *Niemand,* once assigned to Odysseus and is given to know whence they came and *what they want.* Through this very distinction, however, he is already losing ground.

Like the problem of the giving and losing of ground, the problem of fathoming action is pivotal in a play in which the very expanse of the stage comprises a contested territory. At the scene of an unstable peace between two warring armies, Penthesilea, in order to unriddle her actions and her desires, is brought by Achilles to narrate the founding of her nation. The grounds of her actions can only be deduced through the story of their provenance, but – much like the split or doubled origin of Frankenstein's monster – Penthesilea's origin hovers between two disjunct frames: between a mythical explanation and an historical event. When Penthesilea explains to Achilles that she cannot court him but in war, he asks for the origin of the law.

Achilles. Und woher quillt, von wannen ein Gesetz,
Unweiblich, du vergibst mir, unnatürlich,
Dem übrigen Geschlecht der Menschen fremd?
Penthesilea. Fern aus der Urne alles Heiligen,
O Jüngling: von der Zeiten Gipfel nieder,
Den unbetretnen, die der Himmel ewig
In Wolkenduft geheimnisvoll verhüllt. (15.1902-1908)

Achilles
What place, what time could issue such a law,
Unfeminine, forgive me unnatural,
So foreign to all other tribes and nations?
Penthesilea
It issued from the urn of the most holy,
Oh youth: it came from far, from peaks of time,

Untrod by any man, which heaven had
Forever veiled in clouds of mystery. (92)

"Unfeminine, unnatural, foreign to all other tribes," Penthesilea's law, under this unwieldy string of attributes, descends from the shrouded summits of time and issues from a "mother word" held in silence:

Der ersten Mütter Wort entschied es also,
Und dem verstummen wir, Neridensohn,
Wie deiner ersten Väter Worten du.
Achilles. Sei deutlicher. (15.1909-1912)

The word of our first mothers did decree it,
And it commands our silence, son of Thetis,
As your first fathers' word commands your own.
Achilles
Be more specific. (Translation modified, 92.)

But when Achilles demands that she "be more specific," Penthesilea gives an alternate account. In the second account, a more precise genealogy likens the Amazons to "jedwedem andern Volk der Erde" and concludes with the narration of the earthly event that estranged them: an enemy raid followed by capture and enslavement. Achilles describes this, in turn, as the "vernichtendes Schicksal ... das deinem Frauenstaat das Leben gab" (*It was a devastating fate indeed ... that brought your women's state to life* [15.1932-33]).[65] In the second account, the height of time has become the generation of her grandmother; the founding of the state was an act of rebellion. In a final twist, however, when Penthesilea goes on to reveal the origin of the customary removal of the right breast, Achilles exclaims: "Die ungeheure Sage wäre wahr?" "The monstrous legend was true?" (Reese translation, 15.2007) In some sense, then, Achilles has hit upon the speaking mouth of the legendary – Penthesilea offers to decode the mark of tradition on her body, to transcribe myth as history, to embody the history of a myth.

"Mars, an des Schnöden Statt, vollzog die Ehe" (*Mars in his stead carried out the marriage rite)* – this phrase describes the "wedding night" of Tanaïs to the Ethiopian king and the rebellion that was identical to it, recalling Penthesilea's earlier declaration in this same scene: "Er nennt sich marserzeugt, mein Völkerstamm ... " Penthesilea's *nennt sich* is instructive here. The transformation of revolutionary action into a story of origins or, of a foundational act, transpires over the course of one speech. Kleist stages the self-description of a nation that *self-reflectively* knows itself to be naming

65 Note that Achilles finds this story as believable as "Ein Traum, geträumt in Morgenstunden" – fate of the *Dardanenburg*.

itself.[66] The nation comes into being by virtue of the rebellion and simultaneously recasts this generative act into the priority of myth. The instability of this genesis, however, is underscored by the instability of the very scene in which the narration is staged. Achilles' question, after all, derives from the inscrutability of Penthesilea's actions toward him (*Unbegreifliche, wer bist du?*), and the very scene in which she responds to his question is framed by a ruse. Not captive but captor, Penthesilea provides her self-definition to an Achilles who asks under the false pretence of participating in her "ritual," that is, playing the captive by referring to the medieval European idiom of the "captive heart" or "lover's slave."

Alien Nation

> Denn es ist das Los jedes Mythus, allmählich in die Enge einer angeblich historischen Wirklichkeit hineinzukriechen and von irgend einer späteren Zeit als einmaliges Factum mit historischen Ansprüchen behandelt zu werden.
>
> For it is the fate of every myth to creep by degrees into the narrow limits of some alleged historical reality, and to be treated by some later generation as a unique fact with historical claims …
> – Friedrich Nietzsche, *The Birth of Tragedy*

It is possible to argue that with *Penthesilea* Kleist did not contribute to the revisitation of ancient tragedy but entered the ranks of science fiction. One cue for this is the insistence that Odysseus' "nothing third" be a community of self-governing women, freed out of the constraint of the institution of marriage by state-organized reproduction. In *Frankenstein* the Doctor's interruption of women's monopoly on giving birth with his laboratory work poses a dilemma that then presents a whole series of unanswered questions for the articulation of standards for social justice. In *Penthesilea* the state's self-reproduction is answered not with the legal codification of the bourgeouis family but by the Amazonian husband hunt. This "custom" and the exposition of its origin form the "phantasm" of Kleist's *Trauerspiel.* He builds an entire code and mythology which has been taken with remarkable seriousness and literality by many of his readers. Within the imaginary space of this "nation" (which notably calls itself a *Vaterland* and in which the High Priestesses identify themselves as hu-

66 Reading this, one might recall Foucault's question: "Is it not the *Aufklärung*, after all, the first epoch to name itself and, instead of simply characterizing itself, according to an old habit, as a period of decadence or prosperity, of splendor or misery, to name itself after a certain event that comes out of a general history of thought, reason and knowledge, and within which the epoch itself has to play its part?" Foucault, *The Politics of Truth*, 88.

mans, *Menschen*), Kleist's drama enters into the discussion of the so-called Enlightenment of woman (*Aufklärung des Weibes*) of which Goethe's *Iphigenie auf Tauris* is the figure.

With this move, furthermore, Kleist appears to have revisited and revised a position on the "Enlightenment of woman" he had advanced eight years previous in 1800. In a letter addressed to his fiancée, Wilhelmine Zenge, on the subject of religious differences, Kleist confronts the issue of sexual difference for the Enlightenment by embedding the answer in what was just coming to be called "biology" at that time. In addition, the problem of an "Enlightenment for woman" propels Kleist directly into the heart of complexities of cultural translation concomitant to the Colonial era. In the following passage we find our author laboring to produce a formal (notably Kantian) definition of duty that can read transculturally.

> Und doch sind dies alles nur *Zeichen* eines Gefühls, das auch ganz anders sich ausdrücken kann. Denn mit demselben Gefühle, mit welchem Du bei dem Abendmahle das Brot nimmst aus der Hand des Priesters, mit demselben Gefühle, sage ich, erwürgt der Mexikaner seinen Bruder vor dem Altare seines Götzen.
>
> Ich will dich dadurch nur aufmerksam machen, daß alle diese religiösen Gebräuche nichts sind, als *menschliche* Vorschriften, die zu allen Zeiten verschieden waren und noch in diesem Augenblicke an allen Orten der Erde verschieden sind. *Darin* kann das Wesen der Religion nicht liegen, weil es ja sonst höchst schwankend und ungewiß wäre. Wer steht uns dafür, daß nicht in kurzem ein zweiter *Luther* unter uns aufsteht, und umwirft, was jener baute. Aber in uns flammt eine Vorschrift – und die muß göttlich sein, weil sie ewig und allgemein ist; sie heißt: *erfülle Deine Pflicht*; und dieser Satz enthält die Lehren aller Religionen.[67]
>
> And these are all only the *sign* of a feeling, that could also have been expressed very differently. For with the same feeling with which you take communion from the hand of the priest, with the same feeling, I say, the Mexican strangles his brother before the altar of his idol.
>
> I wish only to call to your attention, that all of these religious customs are nothing other than *human* prescriptions, that have been different in all eras and still at this moment are different in all places on earth. The essence of religion cannot lie *therein*, because it were then highly unstable and uncertain. Who can assure us that there will not soon arise a second *Luther* among us to overthrow what the first built? But in us there burns one prescription – and it must be divine, because it is eternal and universal; it runs: *Do your duty*; and this sentence contains the teaching of all religions.[68]

---

67 Heinrich von Kleist, *Sämtliche Werke und Briefe*, vol. 2, 315.

68 Reese translation.

Kleist differentiates between the *Wesen* (essence) of religion and its variant manifestations. He then allies himself with a transcendent concept of religion grounded upon the formal law "fulfill your duty," whatever it may be. The relativity of this Kleistian algebra reaches its own surprising fulfillment in the commanded duty, which issues from his reasoning:

> Deine Bestimmung, liebe Freundin, oder überhaupt die Bestimmung des Weibes ist wohl unzweifelhaft und unverkennbar; denn welche andere kann es sein, als diese, *Mutter zu werden, und der Erde tugendhafte Menschen zu erziehen.*
>
> Und wohl euch, daß eure Bestimmung so einfach und beschränkt ist! Durch euch will die Natur nur ihre Zwecke erreichen, durch uns Männer auch der Staat noch die seinigen, und daraus entwickeln sich oft die unseligsten Widersprüche. (In der Folge mehr.)[69]
>
> This destiny (*Bestimmung*), my dear friend, or the destiny of woman in general is indeed unquestionable and unmistakable; for what other can it be than this, *become a mother, and raise virtuous human beings.*
>
> And happy for you too, that your destiny is so easy and limited! Through you nature only wishes to achieve her ends, while through us men also the state wishes to achieve its ends, and from this the most fatal contradictions often unfold. (More to follow.)[70]

In turning to the question of what duty might be in the case of his fiancée, Kleist answers the question through reference to her *Bestimmung* – determination as one who can become a mother and contribute to the project of *Erziehung*. Further, this *Bestimmung* allows the one *becoming mother* to slip seamlessly into the moral equation through the instrumentalization of her activity as an "end/purpose" of "nature" (*Zweck der Natur*). How to mark out the distance between this "argument" and the drama that includes the speculative concoction of the "Amazon nation?" Likening *Penthesilea* to a syllogism, Kleist wrote to Goethe, "So, wie es hier steht, wird man vielleicht die Prämissen, als möglich, zugeben müssen, und nachher nicht erschrecken, wenn die Folgerung gezogen wird" (*As it is here put forward, one must perhaps accept the premises and then not be horrified when the corollaries are drawn*).

In the letter to Wilhelmine, Kleist shifts Kant's shorthand for enlightenment "the public use of reason" (*der öffentliche Gebrauch der Vernunft*)[71] in his essay "Beantwortung zur Frage: Was heißt Aufklärung" from the singular "use" to the plural "usage," not *Gebrauch* but *Gebräuche.* The discussion of transcendental ethical duty then takes a detour through cultural

69 Ibid., 315.

70 Reese translation.

71 Immanuel Kant, "Was heißt Aufklärung?" in *Schriften zur Anthropologie.*

difference, where ritual sacrifice (located by Kleist somewhere in Mexico) is likened to the differences between Christian denominations in taking communion.[72] The communal importance of the Eucharist and the Mexican sacrifical rite are separated by no more than an ocean. Crossing it, Kleist replies: become a mother (*Mutter werden*) and raise virtuous humans.

But why and how does the "cross cultural" arise as a function of the discussion of the "Enlightenment for woman?" As if the reproductive female body exercised an erosive or dilatory effect on the codes of representation or, indeed, constituted the live point wherein the question of culture begins to feed static into universalizing discourse? It appears that for Kleist in 1800 the issue of biological and cultural reproduction proves itself to be inextricably bound to, yet paradoxically not commensurable with, with Enlightenment ethics. The formal grounding of the law in the command "do your duty" requires the unexpected supplement of a form of natural determination (instrument of a purpose of nature as the unique *Bestimmung* of women). It is worthwhile to note in this context, that Penthesilea does not fail this definition of "Enlightenment" with her customs, but destroys it with her acts. The Amazons are, after all, a nation of enlightened women by Kleist's definition. They become mothers and raise virtuous human beings. Though Kleist does not remark upon the recourse he takes to the problem of cultural difference when addressing the duty of woman, the return of a question concerning the status of women (in the *collective*) in the phantasmatic world of *Penthesilea* written five years later suggests a certain irresolution in the move. Having satisfied the demands of biology with a state-controlled administration of reproduction,[73] *Penthe-*

---

72 Here again, political discussions such as that in the essay contest on the question of Enlightenment correlate with travel narratives and anthropological data gathering of the period. It is by no means clear what Kleist might mean by "the Mexican" in this passage, but the connection between "strangling" and "doing one's duty" suggests that reference is made to ritual sacrifice. As Reinhart Koselleck notes, the confluence of intercontinental travel and the political agitation of the revolutionary may not have been sufficiently accounted for in understanding the period. In a footnote, Koselleck conjectures: "The moral and historico-philosophical significance of the trans-oceanic world was not fully understood in the eighteenth century. The indirect political contribution of the 'outside world' to the shaping of a new society which shattered the Absolutist States has not, as far as I can see, received the scholarly attention it deserves. In its historical sense the 'outside world' of the modern subject is the world beyond Europe. In his 'provisional moral treatise,' Descartes, interestingly enough, compares the outside objects inaccessible to man with China and Mexico (*Discours de la Méthode*, III)" Reinhart Koselleck, *Critique and Crisis: Enlightenment and the Pathogenesis of Modern Society* (New York: Berg Publishers, 1988).

73 Wolf Kittler suggests that Kleist planted a principle of auto-destruction at the core of his fantastic creed of Amazons designed to demonstrate that this woman-society must founder on self-contradiction: "Es führt vor, was geschieht, wenn Frauen all die Dinge tun, die ihrer natürlichen Bestimmung widersprechen: wenn sie freien, wenn sie sich Gesetze ge-

silea presents again the dilemma of the untranslatable, culturally coded fulfillment of duty – a battle between unlike "Nachschriften," between approaches toward the filling-in of variable *x* in the formal moral equation. The tragic drama *Penthesilea* thus returns the question to a battle between these foreign codes, ignoring the efficacy of the the biological determination of women to be reproducers of bodies and educators of children in order to make a crossover possible.

In the essay "'Rights of Man' and 'Rights of the Citizen,' The Modern Dialectic of Equality and Freedom," Balibar elaborates a set of inequalities that he argues cannot be overcome by the institution of equality – in this category he includes sexual difference and the difference between manual and intellectual labor. He writes,

> These two differences thus have in common, negatively, that they are other than inequality, even though they are always inscribed in a relation of power. More precisely they are inscribed in a relation of collective inequality ... which is reproduced, exercised and verified as a personal relation.[74]

The remarkable contribution of the poetics of Kleist's drama derives from the fact that in this later work he is on the case of the particularly unstable and indispensable concept of collective inequalities, which are "reproduced, exercised, and verified" as personal relations. In this work, Kleist seems to locate the crisis in the cultural framing of the gender-sex differential ... at any particular moment. By granting that image production and physical presence can be simultaneous, he allows that the body is a text in a strategic situation. Each move and countermove of perception and of interpretation, each re-alignment of speech and of strategy, reconstellates the way it reads. Like pedestrians who cannot avoid running into each other precisely *because* they are moving out of the way, the attribution of significance to gesture, word or action is caught up in a game that moves faster than any of its players.

> Achilles. Ha! Stellt sie sich? Was bringst du? Stellt sie sich?
> Der Herold. Sie stellt sich, ja Neridensohn, sie naht schon;
> Jedoch mit Hunden auch und Elefanten,

---

ben, wenn sie einen Staat gründen, wenn sie kämpfen. Dabei zeigt sich nicht etwa, daß sie zu alledem unfähig wären, sondern nur, daß es paradoxe Konsequenzen hat, wenn sie diese Dinge tun," Wolf Kittler, *Die Geburt des Partisanen aus dem Geist der Poesie,* 183. The conclusion of Kittler's argument rests on Penthesilea's ultimate renunciation of Amazon-citizenship ("Ich sage mich von dem Gesetze der Frauen los" [24.3012]). He reads the thrice-resounding fall of Penthesilea's bow in repetition of the prophetic "founding fall" of Tanais' bow as signing the death warrant of the Amazon state and signaling the return to a natural order. If one moves temporarily within the fiction of this Amazon state, however, the same instance can be read in opposite fashion, that is, the second fall ratifies the state.

74 Balibar, *Masses, Classes, Ideas,* 55.

Und einem ganzen wilden Reutertroß:
Was beim Zweikampf sollen, weiß ich nicht.
Achilles.
Gut. Dem Gebrauch, war sie das schuldig. Folgt mir!
- O sie ist listig, bei den ewigen Göttern!
- - Mit Hunden, sagst du?
Der Herold. Ja.
Achilles. Und Elefanten? (21.2535-42)

Achilles
Ha! Does she accept? Let's hear it! Does she accept?
Herald
She has, Achilles, yes, she's on her way;
But bringing dogs as well, and elephants,
And a tremendous host of mounted troops;
Why these for single combat, I don't know.
Achilles
That's what she owed the custom. Fine. Now follow!
– Oh she's a sly one, by the eternal gods!
– – With dogs you say?
Herald
Yes, sir.
Achilles
And elephants? (122)

Achilles construes Penthesilea's attack as a ritual and ends his trajectory on Kleist's stage as the sacrifice that Penthesilea deposits at the feet of the High Priestess. Achilles, the heroic anthropologist, moving fast and loose with his newly acquired expertise, is trapped reading significance everywhere without noting that the scene in which he gained it reconditioned the possibilities of signification. He hopes that his insider's knowledge can lead to a mock-up of treaty where unlike principles of war meet. But Penthesilea makes the move to his side, as he passes over to hers, and within the reflection of the attempt: reduplication, collision, and collapse. In this he is fatally transposed into the sheerness of his material presence on stage – de-animated, dead flesh.[75] In the attempt to wed an image to a body – a process expertly executed on the classical stage of Goethe's *Iphigenie* – the center doesn't hold. The significatory system provided by the framing of the stage doesn't superimpose the ideality of the drama upon the physical immediacy of the body argued for in Schiller's concept of the relay between nature and stage effects. Instead, the dramatic figure takes up the stage's "props" (in this case the Amazon body) and re-elaborates them.

75 Penthesilea's description of the Achilles she later finds resonates with the distinction drawn between body and flesh in Hortense J. Spillers riveting article, "Mama's Baby, Papa's Maybe: An American Grammar Book," *Diacritics*, vol. 17, no. 2 (1987), 67-68.

While Achilles' death is, on the one hand, imminently possible despite the long shadow cast by the literary canon produced by the European Humanist tradition, Penthesilea's death is both more and less difficult to execute. Having taken on his unnameable deed – which, true to its immunity to representation, can only take place off stage and be described as an action that has the same effect on the spectator as does the gaze of the Medusa (23.2591-2593) – Penthesilea is left with the task of doubling Achilles again.

Penthesilea. Das aber will ich wissen,
Wer mir so gottlos neben hat gebuhlt! –
Ich frage nicht, wer den Lebendigen
Erschlug; bei unsern ewig hehren Göttern!
Frei, wie ein Vogel, geht er vor mir weg.
Wer mir den Toten tötete, frag ich',
Und darauf gib mir Antwort, Prothoe.
Prothoe. Wie, meine Herrscherin?
Penthesilea. Versteh mich recht.
Ich will nicht wissen, wer aus seinem Busen
Den Funken des Prometheus stahl. Ich will's nicht,
Weil ichs nicht will; die Laune steht mir so:
Ihm soll vergeben sein, er mag entflieh'n.
Doch wer, O Prothoe, bei diesem Raube
Die offne Pforte ruchlos mied, durch alle
Schneeweißen Alabasterwände mir
In diesen Tempel brach; wer diesen Jüngling,
Das Ebenbild der Götter, so entstellt,
Daß Leben und Verwesung sich nicht streiten,
Wem er gehört, wer ihn so zugerichtet,
Daß ihn das Mitleid nicht beweint, die Liebe
Sich, die unsterbliche, bleibt einer Metze,
Im Tod noch untreu, von ihm wenden muß:
Den will ich meiner Rache opfern. Sprich!
Prothoe *zur Oberpriesterin.*
Was soll man nun der Rasenden erwidern? –

Penthesilea
But this I wish to know,
Who courted so godlessly beside me!
I don't ask who the living
Slayed; by our eternal noble gods!
Free, like a bird, he can leave me.
Who killed the dead, I ask
And to this give me an answer, Prothoë.
Prothoë
How was that, my ruler?

Penthesilea

Understand me rightly.
I do not wish to know, who from this breast
stole the spark of Prometheus. I wish it not,
because I don't wish it; such is my whim:
He shall be forgiven, he may run away.
But who, O Prothoë, in the course of this theft,
wickedly scorned the open gate and through all
the snow-white alabaster walls
broke into this temple; who did this youth,
the likeness of the gods, so disfigure,
that Life and Decay no longer vie
to possess him, who so battered him,
that compassion no longer weeps for him, love,
the immortal, like a whore,
in death still untrue, from him must turn:
that one I will sacrifice to my wrath. Speak!

Prothoë (to the High Priestess)

What answer should one give to one who raves? (Reese translation)

Like Sophocles' Oedipus, Penthesilea is looking for herself. At the same time she already transposes the actions committed against Achilles onto herself with the frequent repetition of *mir*, which persistently appropriates the impact of the direct verb in these lines. In one of her last speeches on stage, Penthesilea asks that these actions be narrated to her, for the vision of his desecrated corpse remains mute. Again, Kleist's focus on the possible *generation* of ritual which will follow this scene excludes the necessary conformity of an action to the significance that will be attributed to it. This can only be retrospective, can only be narrated. "This I would like to know" Penthesilea says – tell me. Achilles will not be able to tell, sublimate, embody it. Penthesilea must begin the story herself and does so in this speech when she starts to conjure the alabaster walls and the image of the gate left open.

* * *

Kleist's concern with Kantian ethics interestingly leads him to connect sexual difference with cultural difference. He first binds these by making biological reproduction formally legible so that it can sustain a reference to the status of the not as-yet citizens who bear the potential of becoming mothers (*Mutter werden*) – both biological and cultural reproducers. In renunciation of this reductive answer to the puzzle, however, Kleist's *Penthesilea* remains in motion at the scene of a collision between discourses that might help explain both her unwieldy beauty and her own brand of Frankensteinian fragmentation. *Penthesilea* triggers contradictions in the relay between ideality, in this case in the form of the liberated citizen and the rights for which Iphigenie campaigns, and materiality, the sacrifices and opaque attributes of the culturally coded Amazon body. When Achilles exclaims at the thought of the missing breast, "O Königin!/Der Sitz der jungen, lieblichen Gefühle,/Um eines Wahns, barbarisch – " ("O Queen!/The seat of young, tender feelings,/For a delusion, barbarically – "). Penthesilea parries: "Sei ganz ruhig./Sie retteten in diese Linke sich, Wo sie dem Herzen näher wohnen" ("Be calm./They took refuge in this left breast/Where they live that much closer to the heart"). The peculiar medial quality of Kleist's play disturbs the nascent fusion aroud 1800 of a particular mode of self-reference and the meaning attributed to a body by pointing again and again to the radically generative action of language in dialogue.

For what are the consequences of what I might awkwardly term Penthesilea's status as a subject given these conditions? The preliminary figuration of Penthesilea – first as a kind of weather, second as Odysseus' flat hand – becomes more pointed when the first phase of her inscrutability is connected to the fact that she is the sovereign of a nation that has opted out of marriage. What the Greeks can't grasp is that Penthesilea's body and their desire to represent it cannot be inscribed in terms of the conflict of the Trojan War epic. Rather, the actions of the Amazons are actively refiguring the Greek soldiers as a reserve population. As we finally discover, though Odysseus' keeps asserting that "they must be with us or against," the dizzying onslaught of the Amazons seeks a part resource in assuring their nation's perpetuity. Odysseus thinks they must be allies or enemies, when in fact, his body has been reconstrued as the possible object of capture and use.

Penthesilea oscillates between the two poles either side of the concept of the citizen for the Ancient Greeks: super- or sub-human, she is hero/queen and animal/slave by turns (and each of these couplings include their own differentiation). When the Amazons disavow her at the end of the play, saying she is in the "society of dogs," she is stripped of her Amazon identity though she nevertheless, quite surprisingly, ends the *Trauerspiel* still recognized in her role as ruler. It seems that within the conflict with the Greek soldiers she can be below or above Greek or Amazon law or custom (*Sitte*) but never fully housed within either. The unstable ground across which Penthesilea moves might offer to our reading some sense of the full dimensions of the conflict pointed out by Foucault in the interview "Truth and Power":

> "Dialectic" is a way of evading the always open and hazardous reality of conflict by reducing it to a Hegelian skeleton, and "semiology" is a way of avoid-

> ing its violent, bloody and lethal character by reducing it to the calm Platonic form of language and dialogue.[76]

The dynamic at work in the tragic drama *Penthesilea* insists on the radical contingency of her strategic situation, a situation at the center of which lies the assymetry of a relation of power still open to contest.

Gilles Deleuze and Félix Gauttari offer a reading of the play along the lines of their thinking of the war machine. This reading possesses the unexpected distinction of focusing the elucidation of the "tragic" element in the play on Achilles instead of Penthesilea. Their reading also turns on questions of sovereignty. They find Achilles trapped between two poles of political sovereignty: the outmoded man of war, reduced to his own fury, and the nascent modern State and its representative, Odysseus. It is this same Odysseus who sets Penthesilea outside of the laws of nature. For Deleuze and Guattari's reading, Penthesilea enables Achilles to betray Agamemnon and Odyesseus at the same time.

> In *Penthesilea,* Achilles is already separated from his power: the war machine has passed over to the Amazons, a State-less woman-people whose justice, religion, and loves are organized uniquely in a war mode. Descendants of the Scythians, the Amazons spring forth like lightning, 'between' the two States, the Greek and the Trojan. They sweep away everything in their path. Achilles is brought before his double, Penthesilea. And in his ambiguous struggle, Achilles is unable to prevent himself from marrying the war machine, or from loving Penthesilea, and thus from betraying Agamemnon and Ulysses at the same time.[77]

For my reading, the importance of the role of sovereign in the naming of Penthesilea makes the attribution of the Amazons as "State-less" seem forgetful of one dimension of the play, particularly when one considers the pivotal issue of Penthesilea's status as sovereign at the end. We see elements of this in the above lines in which the appalled Prothoë can no longer recognize her friend but can still recognize "die Herrscherin." Similary, Penthesilea, in a speech meant to shame Meroe for her lack of val-

---

76 Michel Foucault, *Power/Knowledge*, ed. Colin Gordon, trans. Colin Gordon, Leo Marshall, John Mepham, Kate Soper (New York: Pantheon Books, 1980), 114-115.

77 Deleuze and Guattari. *A Thousand Plateaus*, 355. Deleuze and Guattari's understanding of Odysseus seems to take some of its cues from Adorno and Horkheimer's *Dialectic of Enlightenment.*

In James Agee's translation this word has been rendered "Motherland." See Hilda Brown, "Penthesilea: Nightingale and Amazon," *Oxford German Studies* 7 (1973) for a discussion of the importance of the political resonance of the word "Vaterland" in "a period when the ignominy of defeat hung heavy over Prussia" (29). In light of this, translating it as "motherland" significantly blocks access to interpretations trained on the work's political implications.

iance, is notably corrected by her most recent translator when he has her attribute the nation as a "motherland": the word she uses is "Vaterland." The Amazons, who break the "natural law" as Odysseus calls it, are indeed organized under the idea of the "state," the difference is that their state is underived from nature or God. Here also lies their proximity to the monster's attempt in *Frankenstein* to include himself within the frame of the newly declared rights of the eighteenth century. In so doing, the monster has to stand as "particular" and "general" in one body. The single oppositional sexual difference – the sole qualitative difference Kant will admit in his formal definition of the organism at the end of the third *Critique* – immediately pulls a new question of *Gattung* in its train in Kleist's *Penthesilea.* Penthesilea introduces difference in a state form – a particular group that presents a contending locus of sovereignty. Unlike Goethe's Iphigenie, who in the service of producing a universal-as-feminine ethos is the *only woman* on stage, Penthesilea shares the stage with "her kind," who prove ultimately inimical to reconciliation with Odysseus. The Amazons do not make the transition into Odysseus' logic, though their leader takes on new mythic status over the progress of the confrontation.

> Penthesilea. (ein Schauer schüttelt sie zusammen, sie läßt den Bogen fallen)
> Die Oberpriesterin. O die Ensetzliche!
> Prothoe (erschrocken). Nun, was auch gibts?
> Die erste Amazone.
> Der Bogen stürzt ihr aus der Hand danieder!
> Die Zweite.
> Seht, wie er taumelt -
> Die Vierte. Klirrt, und wankt und fällt - !
> Die Zweite. Und noch einmal am Boden zuckt -
> Die Dritte. Und stirbt,
> Wie er der Tanaïs geboren ward.
> (Pause.)
> Die Oberpriesterin. (sich plötzlich zu ihr wendend).
> Du, meine große Herrscherin, vergib mir!
> Diana ist, die Göttin, dir zufrieden,
> Besänftigt wieder hast du ihren Zorn.
> Der große Stifterin des Frauenreiches,
> Die Tanaïs, das gesteh' ich jetzt, sie hat
> Den Bogen würd'ger nicht geführt als du. (24.2768-2775)
>
> [Penthesilea shudders violently; she drops the bow.]
> High Priestess
> Oh the abomination!
> Prothoë (frightened)
> Now what is it?
> First Amazon
> The bow is falling, falling from her hands!

Second Amazon
  Look how it totters –
Fourth Amazon
  Clangs, and sways, and drops – !
Second Amazon
  And shudders one more time upon the ground –
Third Amazon
  And dies – as it was born to Queen Tanaïs.
  [Pause]
High Priestess
  (suddenly turning to Penthesilea)
  Oh my great Queen and mistress, please forgive me!
  Well pleased is Artemis, the goddess, with you,
  Your deed has put her anger back to rest.
  The mighty founder of our women's state,
  Tanaïs herself, I will admit it now,
  Wielded the bow no worthier than you. (133-34)

The priestess' sudden turn in this scene recuperates the nameless Penthesilea back into the Amazon fold under the terms of her office of state: "große Herrscherin." Unlike Iphigenie, who talks herself out of one mythological status and office of duty into another to become the enlightened brother's sister and father's daughter of Goethe's stage, Penthesilea, almost fatally transposed into Achilles' courtly language, reaches the end of Kleist's drama a mythically inflected figure the High Priestess can no longer judge. While Iphigenie speaks a new law into being, Penthesilea ends the play in abrogation of the law, restored as sovereign and re-mythified – a process we have observed with the slow, silent series of gestures we witness as she regains consciousness. Close attention to the last scene of Kleist's *Trauerspiel* should affirm its *hope* for an eventual performance. The corpse on stage, victim of violence, *becomes* a sacrifice through the ceremony of its placement and the rage of the personage who has destroyed a citadel they had wished to found. Once more, a powerful reflection upon the status of body, object and speech on stage.

Penthesilea follows Achilles into his death, or rather the death of his death, not mirroring, but transposed onto the violation of his body's social promise. She follows him, tracing as she goes those other movements that shadow the figures on stage, the bodies which flee and are pursued by names.

Exposed, in the Vibration of the Word

One might recall Antonin Artaud's statement in "Metaphysics and the Mise en Scène": "And what the theater can still take over from speech are its possibilities for extension beyond words, for development in space, for dissociative and vibratory action upon the sensibility."[78] If *Penthesilea*'s stage watches the refiguration and disappearance of a mythic body threatened by elucidation (Greek anthropology), as theater it releases words that don't so much "express" as produce dissociative effects. The high-speed movements that constitute the battle for the stage boards in *Penthesilea*, could also trace out the possibility for a theater Artaud proposes, when he asserts, "The theater still remains the most active and efficient *site of passage* for those immense analogical disturbances in which ideas are arrested in flight at some point in their transmutation into the abstract."[79] It is not the full reconciliation of particular and general that Kleist captures but rather the flight between the two – and *that* as a battle, a conflict, a chase. In this sense, he could also be said to put radical use to the screen which classical German aesthetics was making of *Einbildungskraft*.[80]

That Kleist chose a classical myth with only fragmentary antecedents points to the possibility that *Penthesilea* includes the historical present within the scope of the "classical." Both the invention of an Amazon state and that state's self-exposition reflect upon new or invented "founding mythologies" and their relation to productions of the stage. In this, the play also directly intervenes in the scene of Enlightenment Europe's willed designation of Greek antiquity as its rightful ancestor in the universally human. Rather than preparing the ideality of nature, as Schiller would have it in his discussion of the chorus in *Die Braut von Messina*, Kleist's theater, almost like a developing agent, brings out ideality *alongside* nature, that is, a disjunctive coexistence of ascriptions, actions, bodies, and desires. The embedded structure of conflict which organizes the drama at

78 Antonin Artaud, "Metaphysics and the Mise en Scène" in *The Theater and its Double*, trans. Mary Caroline Richards (New York: Grove Press, 1958), 89.

79 Ibid., 109.

80 Though Kleist's dramas are so word-riddled that, in some cases, as in *Penthesilea*, they barely comprise any action other than speakers taking possession of the stage, they were also decried as "circuses" by their contemporaries as noted in an earlier section of this chapter. It is in their spectacular, if merely linguistic, enormity that they are consonant with Artaud's conjurations. As for instance in "The Theater and Cruelty," where Artaud writes, "Practically speaking, we want to resuscitate an idea of total spectacle by which the theater would recover from the cinema, the music hall, the circus and from life itself what has always belonged to it" (Artaud, *The Theater and its Double*, 86). The values and distinctions of the written text take over the stage, but they are as easily swept off by the magnetic forces the words begin to exert on one another, dislocating them from their wonted purposes or, otherwise, bringing their sedimentation to light. This is also the case with Penthesilea who with the same destructive potency that Artaud attributes to the true meaning of comedy is released into a flight and not a resolution of metaphors – from figures of speech further to a flight of forms. "Wie Sturmwind ein zerrissenes Gewölk ... " (I., 35) ("Like a high-wind from torn clouds...").

the level of its action disrupts various models of perception, identity formation, and codes of recognition. In some instances, even a repetition becomes a translation, a word transposed into an altered landscape.

In the first decade of the nineteenth century, Kleist introduced a play that could only be staged *in potentia*, that had no predecessor among extant ancient Greek tragedies and that took up, to use Kleist's word "the gruesome riddle" (*das Greuelrätsel*) that motivates the denouement of Homer's *Iliad*. Who killed the dead? Who added to the rigors of combat the violence against custom? Hector's tortured corpse is joined by that of Achilles' at the end of Kleist's contribution to Weimar Classicism. Kleist seems to be threatening to pull new German literature out by its roots.

Epilogue

This book began with a note taken in the margins of Roland Barthes essay, "Is There Any Poetic Writing?" Looking back, I see the sentence reads:

> In modern poetics, on the contrary, words produce a kind of formal continuum from which there gradually emanates an intellectual or emotional density which would have been impossible without them; speech is then the solidified time of a more spiritual gestation, during which the 'thought' is prepared, installed little by little by the contingency of words.[1]

Where in Barthes' view classical thought is "devoid of duration," the work he calls modern forges the relation between language and thought contingently, in time. Beside this remarkable passage I wrote "Kleist." Though it was not only the more apparent connection to "On the Gradual Formulation of Thoughts while Speaking" that led me to do so, but something about the verse that accompanies Penthesilea's return to consciousness in captivity, in the 14th Scene of Kleist's play.

> Ich war so ruhig, Prothoe, wie das Meer,
> Das in der Bucht des Felsen liegt; nicht ein
> Gefühl, das sich in Wellen mir erhob.
> Dies Wort: sei ruhig! jagt mich plötzlich jetzt,
> Wie Wind die offnen Weltgewässer auf.
> Was ist es denn, das Ruh hier nötig macht? - (14.1586-91)

> I was as calm, Prothoe, as the sea
> that lies in the cove between the cliffs; not one
> Feeling, in waves, in me arose.
> These words, "Be calm!" chase me suddenly now
> Like wind across the oceans' waters.
> What is it, then, that here makes calm a need?[2]

Penthesilea's speech bears witness to a contest that runs the race for meaning and the vectors of power from within which words emerge. It is thus that Penthesilea "answers with arrows" or Meroe, an Amazon messenger, names herself the Gorgon Medusa when she undertakes to re-

1 Roland Barthes, trans. Annette Lavers and Colin Smith, *Writing Degree Zero* (New York: Hill and Wang, 1994), 43.

2 Reese translation.

count her sovereign's incomprehensible acts. "This Hunger of the Word, common to the whole of modern poetry, makes poetic speech terrible and inhuman."[3] It was with a fascination for the terrible and inhuman in the first decades of the 19th century that this project took shape. First as a quest after Kleist's poetry and the possibility that in it "[E]ach poetic word is an unexpected object, a Pandora's box from which fly out all the potentialities of language." [4]

At the same time, I wanted to track the consolidation of the category of the self-evident in the name of the human taking shape in the period from which Kleist's lyric took flight. For though the Kleistian word was avowedly becoming object, the ideas of culture around it were rather coming into a living and sensuous immediacy that bespoke a secularizing world shearing itself gradually of all the "dead tokens" of allegory. I became interested in how the "terrible and inhuman" also reveals the way in which members of distinct collectivities and members of the "same" collectivity might fall away from the forms of self-evidence underwriting political legibility and legitimacy. Reproduction presented a category which could reveal sedimentation in those words "self-evident."

Between two literary readings, I have undertaken a reading of Kant's bridge, *Critique of Judgment.* Kant insists that judgment must be practiced, must take place in time, even as his critique seeks passages back out of time, away from the contingent and toward the universal. I read Kant to learn about the formation of an understanding of the organism that will increasingly prepare the possibility for something like "cultural history"– the idea that beings, in their material form, could self-sufficiently reflect and thereby represent themselves, universally, or even more interestingly become signs of their own being *in becoming.* I have contrasted this idea with a modern poetics which temporizes with language's polyphony and makes a profound inquiry into the problems which emerge in strategies for universal and teleological designations. In so doing this poetics reintroduces the allegorical dimension to literary language even as Romantic era thinkers and poets are sounding its demise.

From these spurs emerged a comparative reading of Mary Shelley's *Frankenstein: A Modern Prometheus* and Kleist's *Penthesilea.* For, Shelley's novel too insists importantly on the contingencies of its own becoming-in-time, the forces of narrative concatenation in this novel which starkly contrast with the compelling claim voiced by the unnameable monster who bursts its frame. The protagonist of each equally "inhuman," and

3 Ibid., 48.

4 Ibid.

equally descended from doubled, fraught and unstable origins, these two works of literature admit of a reconsideration of the possibilities contained within Enlightenment fictions of origins and their importance to the modern expansion of the discourse on natural law. They look to the paradoxes of origins in attempts to think justice around 1800 as distinct and separable from the labor of the domestic and economic spheres.

Among the outcomes of my investigation, one is that it is not "nature" that divides the non-citizen from the law in "natural law" but rather asymmetries in social relations which can never be confronted solely in terms of a formal equality. Rather, material force will exert its toll on the intelligible, and here, politically, aesthetically and culturally, the fight is waged for recognition in difference. This struggle keeps literature, keeps language, on the move, in flux. If Kleist's *Penthesilea* shakes up the hope to found an essential human being in the idea of culture as singular universal, preferring instead the volatility and risk of contingent, never univocal, nor necessarily commensurable meaning, then it could inspire us students and producers of culture to avoid the monolith presented in this word and its false placidity.

Works Cited

Adorno, Theodor W. "Zum Klassizismus von Goethe's Iphigenie." In *Noten zur Literatur*. Frankfurt am Main: Suhrkamp, 1979.

---. *Notes to Literature*. Translated by Shierry Weber Nicholsen. New York: Columbia University Press, 1992.

---. *Problems of Moral Philosophy*. Translated by Rodney Livingstone. Stanford: Stanford University Press, 2001.

Adorno, Theodor W. and Horkheimer, Max. *Dialektik der Aufklärung: Philosophische Fragmente*. Frankfurt am Main: Fischer, 1994.

---. *Dialectic of Enlightenment: Philosophical Fragments*. Translated by Edmund Jephcott. Stanford: Stanford University Press, 2002.

Allison, Henry. *Kant's Theory of Freedom*. New York: Cambridge University Press, 1990.

Althusser, Louis. *Montesquieu, Rousseau, Marx*. Translated by Ben Brewster. London: verson, 1982.

---. *Lenin and Philosophy and Other Essays*. Translated by Ben Brewster. New York: Monthly Review Press, 2001.

Angress, Ruth. "Kleist's Nation of Amazons." In *Beyond the Eternal Feminine: Critical Essays on Women and German Literature*, 101-7. Stuttgart: Akademischer Verlag Hans-Dieter Heinz, 1982.

Arendt, Hannah. *The Origins of Totalitarianism*. New York: Harcourt, Brace and World, 1966.

---. *Lectures on Kant's Political Philosophy*. Edited by Ronald Beiner. Chicago: University of Chicago Press, 1982.

Artaud, Antonin. "Metaphysics and the Mise-en-Scène." In *The Theater and its Double*. Translated by Mary Caroline Richards. New York: Grove Press, 1958.

Aspen Municipal Code. §§13-98(b),(c). 1977.

Austin, J.L. *How to Do Things with Words*. Cambridge: Harvard University Press, 1975.

Balibar, Etienne. *Masses, Classes, Ideas*. Translated by James Swenson. New York: Routledge, 1994.

---. *Politics and the Other Scene.* Translated by Christine Jones. New York: Verso, 2002.

Bacon, Francis. *Francis Bacon.* Edited by Arthur Johnson. New York: Schocken Books, 1965.

Baldick, Chris. "The Politics of Monstrosity." In *New Casebooks: Frankenstein*, ed. Fred Botting. New York: MacMillan, 1995.

Barthes, Roland. *Writing Degree Zero.* Translated by Annette Lavers and Colin Smith. New York: Hill and Wang, 1994.

Beckett, Samuel. *Ends and Odds.* London: Faber & Faber, 1977.

Benjamin, Walter. *Gesammelte Schriften.* 14 vols. Frankfurt am Main: Suhrkamp, 1977.

---. *The Origin of German Tragic Drama.* Translated by John Osbourne. London: NLB, 1977.

---. *Reflections: Essays, Aphorisms, Autobiographical Writings.* Translated by Edmund Jephcott. New York: Harcourt Brace Jovanovich, 1978.

---. *New Left Review* I/133 (1982).

Bloch, Ernst. *Naturrecht und menschliche Würde.* Frankfurt am Main: Suhrkamp, 1961.

---. *Natural Law and Human Dignity.* Translated by Dennis J. Schmidt. Cambridge: MIT Press, 1986.

Blumenbach, Johann Friedrich. *Über den Bildungstrieb (Nisus formativus) und seinen Einfluss auf die Generation und Reproduction.* Göttingen, 1789.

Botting, Fred. *Making Monstrous: Frankenstein, Criticism, Theory.* Manchester: Manchester University Press, 1991.

---. "Reflections of Excess: *Frankenstein*, the French Revolution and Monstrosity." In *Reflections of Revolution: Images of Romanticism.* Edited by Alison Yarrington and Kelvin Everest. London and New York: Routledge, 1993.

Boulder Rev. Code §§12-1-2, 12-1-3. 1987.

Brandstetter, Gabrielle, and Gerhard Neumann. "Opferfest – Sacre du Printemps." In *Konflikt, Grenze, Dialog: Kulturkontrastive und interdisziplinäre Textzugänge.* Frankfurt am Main: Peter Lang, 1997.

Brooks, Peter. "What is a Monster?" In *New Casebooks: Frankenstein.* Edited by Fred Botting. London: MacMillan, 1995.

Butler, Judith. *Gender Trouble: The Subversion of Identity.* New York: Routledge, 2006.

---. *Antigone's Claim: Kinship Between Life and Death.* New York: Columbia University Press, 2002.

Butler, Judith, and Spivak, Gayatri Chakravorty. *Who Sings the Nation State.* Calcutta: Seagull Books, 2007.

Campe, Rüdiger. *Spiel der Wahrscheinlichkeit: Literatur und Rechnung zwischen Pascal und Kleist.* Göttingen: Wallstein, 2002.

Carson, James P. "Bringing the Author Forward: *Frankenstein* through Mary Shelley's Letters." In *Criticism* 30, no. 4 (1988): 431-53.

Caruth, Cathy. *Empirical Truths and Critical Fictions: Locke, Wordsworth, Kant, Freud.* Baltimore: Johns Hopkins University Press, 1991.

Cassirer, Ernst. *Rousseau, Goethe, Kant.* Translated by James Gultman, Paul Oskar Kristeller and John Hermann Randall, Jr. Princeton: Princeton University Press, 1945.

---. *Kant's Life and Thought.* Translated by James Haden. New Haven: Yale University Press, 1981.

Condillac, Etienne Bonnot de. *Essay on the Origin of Human Knowledge.* Edited by Hans Aarsleff. Cambridge: Cambridge University Press, 2001.

Cullins, Chris and Mücke, Dorothea E. von. "Love in Kleist's *Penthesilea* and *Käthchen von Heilbronn.*" In *Deutsche Vierteljahrsschrift für Literaturwissenschaft und Geistesgeschichte*, 63, no. 3 (1989).

Deleuze, Gilles. *Kant's Critical Philosophy.* Translated by Hugh Tomlinson and Barbara Habberjam. Minneapolis: University of Minnesota Press, 1984.

Deleuze, Gilles and Guattari, Félix. *A Thousand Plateaus.* Translated by Brian Massumi. Minneapolis: University of Minnesota Press, 1987.

Derrida, Jacques. "Déclarations d'indépendence." In *Otobiographies: l'enseignement de Nietzsche et la politique du nom propre.* Paris: Gallimard, 1984.

---. *The Truth in Painting.* Translated by Geoff Bennington and Ian McLeod. Chicago: University of Chicago Press, 1987.

---. "Force of Law." In *Deconstruction and the Possibility of Justice.* Edited by Drucilla Cornell et al. New York: Routledge, 1992.

Engel, Johann Jakob. *Ideen zu einer Mimik.* Berlin, 1786.

Fink, Karl J. "Kant's Concept of Telos: Reviews Shaping Anthropology." In *The Eighteenth Century Book Review.* Edited by Herbert Rowland and Karl J. Fink, 169-80. Heidelberg: Universitätsverlag, 1995.

Fischer-Lichte, Erika. *Theater im Prozeß der Zivilisation.* Tübingen: Franke, 2000.

---. "Theatralität: Zur Frage nach Kleists Theaterkonzeption." In *Kleist Jahrbuch 2001*. Stuttgart: Verlag J.B. Metzler, 2001.

Förster, Eckart. *Kant's Final Synthesis.* Cambridge: Harvard University Press, 2000.

---. "Die Bedeutung von §§76, 77 von Kants *Kritik der Urteilskraft* für die Entwicklung der nachkantischen Philosophie." In *Zeitschrift für philosophische Forschung*, Band 56 (2002).

Foucault, Michel. *The History of Sexuality: An Introduction*, Vol. 1. Translated by Robert Hurley. New York: Random House, 1978.

---. *Power/Knowledge.* Edited by Colin Gordon. Translated by Colin Gordon, Leo Marshall, John Mepham and Kate Soper. New York: Panteon Books, 1980.

---. *The Politics of Truth.* Edited by Sylvère Lotringer. New York: Semiotext(e), 1997.

Freeman, Barbara Claire. "*Frankenstein* with Kant: A Theory of Monstrosity or the Monstrosity of Theory." In *New Casebooks: Frankenstein.* Edited by Fred Botting. London: MacMillan, 1995.

Gallas, Helga. "Kleists *Penthesilea* und Lacans vier Diskurse." In *Kontroversen, alte und neue. Akten des VII Kongresses der Internationalen Vereinigung der germanistischen Sprach- und Literaturwissenschaft.* Edited by Albrecht Schöne. Tübingen, 1986.

Gay, Peter. *The Enlightenment: The Rise of Modern Paganism.* New York: W.W. Norton, 1995.

Genette, Girard. *Palimpsests: Literature in the Second Degree.* Lincoln: University of Nebraska Press, 1997.

Ginsborg, Hannah. "Two Kinds of Mechanical Inexplicability in Kant and Aristotle." In *Journal of the History of Philosophy* 42 (1): 33-65.

---. "Kant's Biological Teleology and its Philosophical Significance." In *Blackwell Companion to Kant.* Edited by Graham Bird. Oxford: Blackwell Publishing, 2006, 455-69.

Girard, René. *Violence and the Sacred.* Translated by Patrick Gregory. Baltimore: Johns Hopkins University Press, 1977.

Goethe, Johann Wolfgang von. *Goethe's Plays.* Translated by Charles E. Passage. New York: Frederick Ungar Publishing Co., 1980.

---. *Goethe: The Collected Works*. Edited by John Grearey. Translated by Ellen von Nardoff and Ernest H. von Nardoff. New York: Suhrkamp Publishers, 1986.

---. *Sämtliche Werke*. Frankfurt am Main: Deutscher Klassiker Verlag, 1988.

Hansen, Mark. "Parody of Romantic Poetics in *Frankenstein*." In *SiR* 36 (1997): 575-609.

Hederich, Benjamin. *Gründliches Mythologisches Lexikon*. Darmstadt: Wissenschaftliche Buchgesellschaft, 1996.

Hegel, Georg Wilhelm Friedrich. *Phenomenology of Spirit*. Translated by A. V. Miller. New York: Oxford University Press, 1977.

---. *Philosophy of Right*. Translated by Alan White. Newburyport: Focus Philosophical Library, 2002.

Heidegger, Martin. *Kant and the Problem of Metaphysics*. Translated by Richard Taft. Bloomington: Indiana University Press, 1990.

Hohendahl, Peter. *Prismatic Thought*. Lincoln: University of Nebraska Press, 1997.

---. *Literary Paternity, Literary Friendship*, ed. Gerhard Richter. Chapel Hill: University of North Carolina, 2002.

Horst, Falk. "Kleists Penthesilea oder die Unfähigkeit aus Liebe zu kämpfen." In *Germanisch-Romanische Monatsschrift* 36, no. 2 (1986): 150-68.

Jacobs, Carol. *Uncontainable Romanticism: Shelley, Brontë, Kleist*. Baltimore: Johns Hopkins University Press, 1989.

Johnson, Barbara. "My Monster/My Self." In *Diacritics* 12, no. 2 (1982): 2-10.

Kant, Immanuel. *Kritik der reinen Vernunft*. Leipzig: Verlag von Feliz Meiner, 1930.

---. *Critique of Pure Reason*. Translated by Werner S. Pluhar. Indianapolis: Hackett, 1996.

---. *Schriften zur Naturphilosophie*. Edited by Wilhelm Weischedel. Frankfurt am Main: Suhrkamp, 1968.

---. *Werkausgabe*. 12 vols. Edited by Wilhelm von Weischedel. Frankfurt am Main: Suhrkamp, 1974.

---. *Prolegomena to Any Future Metaphysics that Will be Able to Come Forward as a Science*. Translated by Paul Carus, extensively revised by James W. Ellington. In *Philosophy of Material Nature*. Indianapolis: Hackett, 1985.

---. "Metaphyscial Foundations of Natural Science." In *Immanuel Kant: Philosophy of Nature*. Indianapolis: Hackett, 1985.

---. *Critique of Judgment*. Translated by Werner S. Pluhar. Indianapolis: Hackett, 1987.

---. *Prolegomena zu einer jeden künftigen Metaphysik, die als Wissenschaft wird auftreten können*. Erlangen: Fischer, 1988.

---. *Critique of Pure Reason*. Translated by Paul Guyer. Cambridge: Cambridge University Press, 1988.

---. *Political Writings*. Edited by Hans Reiss. Cambridge: Cambridge University Press, 1991.

---. *Critique of Practical Reason*. Translated by Lewis White Beck. New Jersey: Prentice Hall, 1993.

---. *The Metaphysics of Morals*. Translated by Mary J. Gregor. New York: Cambridge University Press, 1996.

---. *Foundations of the Metaphysics of Morals and What is Enlightenment?* Translated by Lewis White Beck. New Jersey: Prentice Hall, 1997.

---. *Religion within the Boundaries of Mere Reason*. Edited and translated by Allen Wood and George di Giovani. New York: Cambridge University Press, 1998.

Ketterer, David. "The Corrected *Frankenstein*: Twelve Preferred Readings in the Last Draft." In *English Language Notes* 33, no. 1 (1995): 23-35.

---. "(De)Composing *Frankenstein*: The Import of Altered Character Names in the Last Draft." In *Studies in Bibliography: Papers of the Bibliographical Society of the University of Virginia*49 (1996): 232-76.

Kittler, Wolf. *Geburt des Partisanen aus dem Geist der Poesie*. Freiburg im Breisgau: Rombach Verlag, 1987.

Kleist, Heinrich. *Sämtliche Werke und Briefe*. 2 vols. Edited by Hans Rudolf Barth et al. Frankfurt am Main: Deutscher Klassiker Verlag, 1987.

---. *Penthesilea: A Tragic Drama*. Translated by Joel Agee. New York: Harper Collins, 1998.

Klotz, Volker. "Aug um Zunge – Zunge um Aug, Kleists extremes Theater." In *Kleist Jahrbuch* (1985): 128-42.

Kosch, Michelle. *Freedom and Reason in Kant, Schelling and Kiekegaard*. Oxford: Clarendon Press, 2006.

Koselleck, Reinhart. *Futures Past: On the Semiotics of Historical Time*. Cambridge: MIT Press, 1985.

---. *Critique and Crisis: Enlightenment and the Pathogenesis of Modern Society.* New York: Berg Publishers, 1988.

Kosenina, Alexander. "Will er 'auf ein Theater warten, welches da kommen soll?.'" In *Kleist Jahrbuch 2001.* Stuttgart: Verlag J.B. Metzler, 2001.

Lehman, Hans-Thies. "Kleist/Versionen." In *Kleist Jahrbuch 2001.* Stuttgart: Verlag J.B. Metzler, 2001.

Lem, Stanislaw. *Solaris.* Krakow: Wydawn Literackie, 1994.

Lenoir, Timothy. *The Strategy of Life: Teleology and Mechanics in Nineteenth-Century German Biology.* Studies in the History of Modern Science, vol. 13. Boston: Kluwer Boston, 1982.

Lepenies, Wolf. *Das Ende der Naturgeschichte: Wandel kultureller Selbstverständlichkeiten in den Wissenschaften des 18. und 19. Jahrhunderts.* Munich: Carl Hanser Verlag, 1976.

Lévi-Strauss. *Tristes Tropiques.* Translated by John and Doreen Weightman. New York: Atheneum, 1977

London, Bette. "Mary Shelley's *Frankenstein* and the Spectacle of Masculinity." *PMLA* 108 (1993): 253-67.

Marx, Karl. "On the Jewish Question." In *The Marx-Engels Reader*, 2nd edition. Edited by Robert C. Tucker. New York: W.W. Norton, 1978.

---. "Zur Judenfrage." in vol. 1 of *Philosophie: Studienausgabe.* Edited by Fetscher. Frankfurt am Main: Fischer Taschenbush Verlag, 1990.

Miller, Hillis J. *Versions of Pygmalion.* Cambridge: Harvard University Press, 1990.

Müller-Seidel, Walter. *Versehen und Erkennen: Eine Studie über Heinrich von Kleist.* Cologne: Böhlau, 1961.

---. *Die Geschichtlichkeit der deutschen Klassik: Literatur und Denkformen um 1800.* Stuttgart: Metzlersche Verlagsbuchhandlung, 1983.

Müller-Sievers, Helmut. *Self-Generation: Biology, Philosophy and Literature around 1800.* Stanford: Stanford University Press, 1997.

Newman, Beth. "The Frame Structure of *Frankenstein.*" In *New Casebooks: Frankenstein.* Edited by Fred Botting. London: MacMillan Press, 1995.

Oellers, Norbert, and Robert Steegers, eds. *Treffpunk Weimar.* Stuttgart: Reclam, 1999.

O'Flinn, Paul. "Production and Reproduction: the Case of *Frankenstein*." In *The Study of Popular Fiction*. Edited by Bob Ashley, 23-29. London: Printer Publishers, 1989.

O'Rourke, James. "'Nothing More Unnatural': Mary Shelley's Revision of Rousseau." In *ELH* 56, 1989.

Pateman, Carole. *The Sexual Contract*. Cambridge: Polity Press, 1988.

Pfeiffer, Joachim. "Kleists 'Penthesilea' Eine Deutung unter den Aspekten von narzißtischer und ödipaler Problematik." In *Kontroversen alte und neue: Akten des III Internationalen Germanistischen Kongresses*. Edited by Albrecht Schöne. Göttingen, 1985.

Poovey, Mary. "My Hideous Progeny: Mary Shelley and the Feminization of Romanticism. In *PMLA* 95 (1980): 332-47.

Rousseau, Jean-Jacques. *Ouevres complètes*. 4 vols. Dijon: Éditions Gallimard (Pléiade), 1959.

---. *Reveries of the Solitary Walker*. Translated by Peter France. New York: Penguin Classics, 1979.

---. *The First and Second Discourses*. Translated by Victor Gourevitch. New York: Perennial Library, 1986.

Schiller, Friedrich. "On the Use of the Chorus in Tragedy." In *The Bride of Messina, William Tell, Demetrius*. Translated by Charles E. Passage. New York: Frederick Ungar Publishing, 1962.

---. *Werke und Briefe*. 12 vols. Frankfurt am Main: Deutscher Klassiker Verlag, 1992.

Schneider, Manfred. "Die Welt im Ausnahmezustand." In *Kleist Jahrbuch 2001*. Stuttgart: Verlag J.B. Metzler, 2001.

Schoene-Harwood, Berthold, ed. *Mary Shelley: Frankenstein*. New York: Columbia University Press, 2000.

Semdner, Helmut, ed. *Heinrich von Kleists Lebensspuren: Dokumente und Berichte der Zeitgenossen*. Munich: Hanser, 1996.

---. *Heinrich von Kleists Nachruhm: Eine Wirkungsgeschichte in Dokumenten*. Munich: Hanser, 1996.

Shelley, Mary. *Frankenstein, or, The Modern Prometheus*. In *Three Gothic Novels*, ed. Peter Fairclough. New York: Penguin, 1988.

---. *The Novels and Selected Works of Mary Shelley*. Edited by Nora Crook and Pamela Clemit. London: W. Pickering, 1996.

Sherwin, Paul. "*Frankenstein*: Creation as Catastrophe." In *PMLA* 96 (1981): 883-903.

Sørensen, Bengt Algot. "Die zarte Differenz." In *Formen und Funktionen der Allegorie*. Edited by Walter Haug. Stuttgart: J.B. Metzlersche, 1979.

Spillers, Hortense. "Mama's Baby, Papa's Maybe: An American Grammar Book." In *Diacritics*, 17, no. 2 (1987): 64-81.

Spivak, Gayatri Chakravorty. *A Critique of Postcolonial Reason*. Cambridge: Harvard University Press, 1999.

Stafford, Barbara Maria. *Body Criticism: Imaging the Unseen in Enlightenment Art and Medicine*. Cambridge: MIT Press, 1991.

Starobinski, Jean. *Jean-Jacques Rousseau: la transparence et l'obstacle*. Paris: Gallimard, 1971.

Sterne, Laurence. *Tristram Shandy*. New York: W.W. Norton, 1980.

Sterrenburg, Lee. "Mary Shelley's Monster: Politcs and Psyche in *Frankenstein*." In *The Endurance of Frankenstein*, ed. George Levin and U.C. Knoepflmacher. Berkeley: University of California Press, 1979.

Stollberg-Rilinger, Barbara. *Europa im Jahrhundert der Aufklärung*. Stuttgart: Reclam, 2000.

Szondi, Peter. *An Essay on the Tragic*. Translated by Paul Fleming. Stanford: Stanford University Press, 2002.

Vernant, Jean-Pierre, and Vidal-Naquet, Pierre. *Myth and Tragedy in Ancient Greece*. New York: Zone Books, 1988.

Wall, Richard, Jareven, Tamara K. and Ehmer, Joseph, eds. *Family History Revisited: Comparative Perspectives*. Newark: University of Delaware Press, 2001.

Yovel, Yiramiahu. *Kant and the Philosophy of History*. Princeton: Princeton University Press, 1980.

Zammito, John H. *The Genesis of Kant's Critique of Judgment*. Chicago: Chicago University Press, 1992.

Zizek, Slavoj. "Why Does the Law Need an Obscene Supplement?" In *Law and the Postmodern Mind: essays on Psychoanalysis and Jursiprudence*. Edited by Peter Goodrich and David Gray Carlson. Ann Arbor: University of Michigan Press, 1998.

Index